Vitamins! A Colorful Grocery Trip

Vertex Wellness, LLC.

Vitamins!/Dr. Brandon D. Beamon – 978-1-7368840-1-0

Pages:

https://www.drdeanbeamon.com/

https://www.linkedin.com/in/brandon-beamon-ph-d-23049016a/

https://speakerhub.com/speaker/brandon-beamon

Attention

The author made every effort to be as precise and thorough as possible while crafting this book. Even though the author does not warrant or represent at any time that the content is accurate due to the rapidly ever-changing internet and sources. Citations were utilized during the writing process to be presented to the reader for further education. All efforts have been meticulously made to confirm the information presented in this publication. The author assumes no responsibility and is not liable for errors, omissions, or contrary interpretations of the subject matter in the text. The author hereby denies any liability, loss or damage incurred due to the use and utilization, whether directly or indirectly, of any information, suggestion, or advice in this literary work. **Please see a registered dietician, pediatrician, or primary care doctor for your specific health needs.**

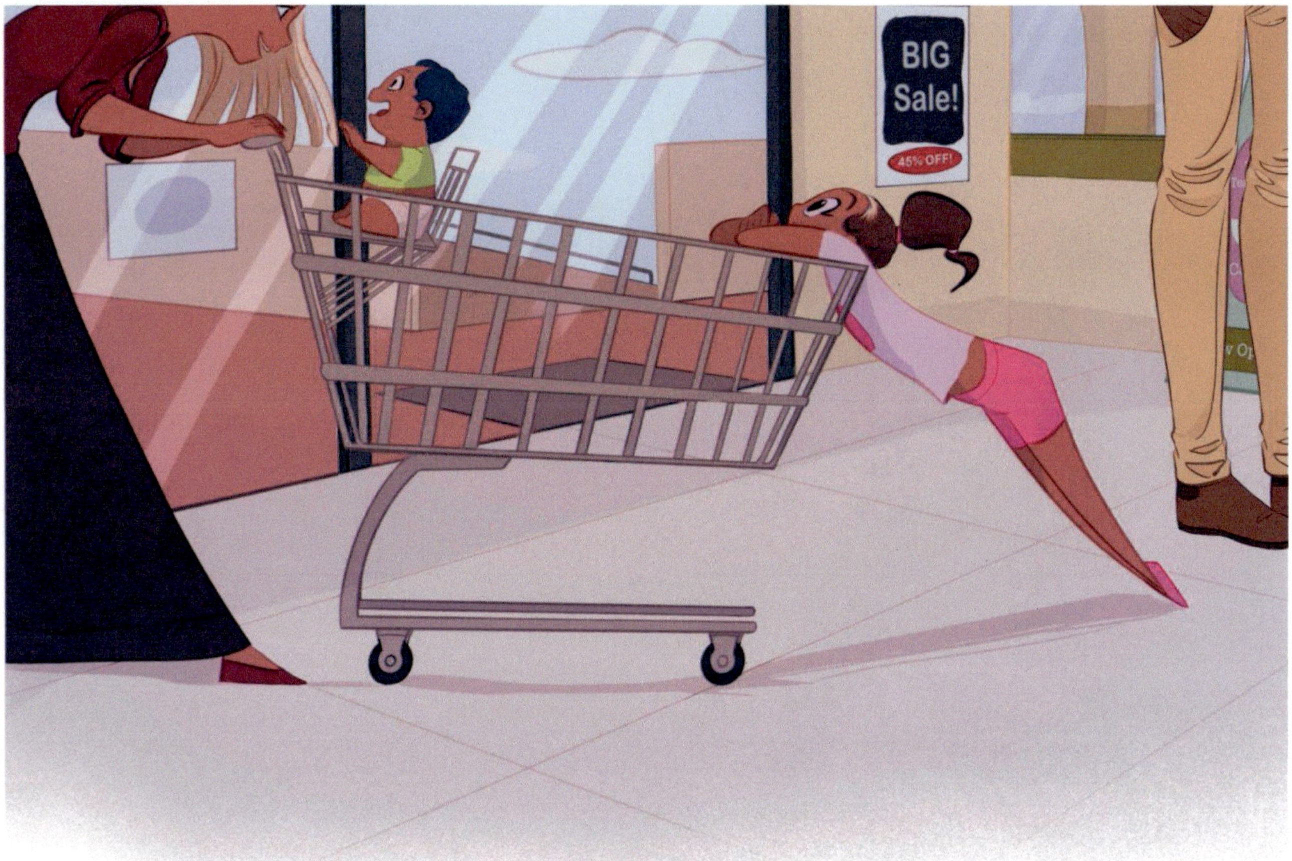

A family of four goes to the store.
Bro and sis want to fill the bins.

Mom and dad put on a grin; And
introduced them to vitamins.

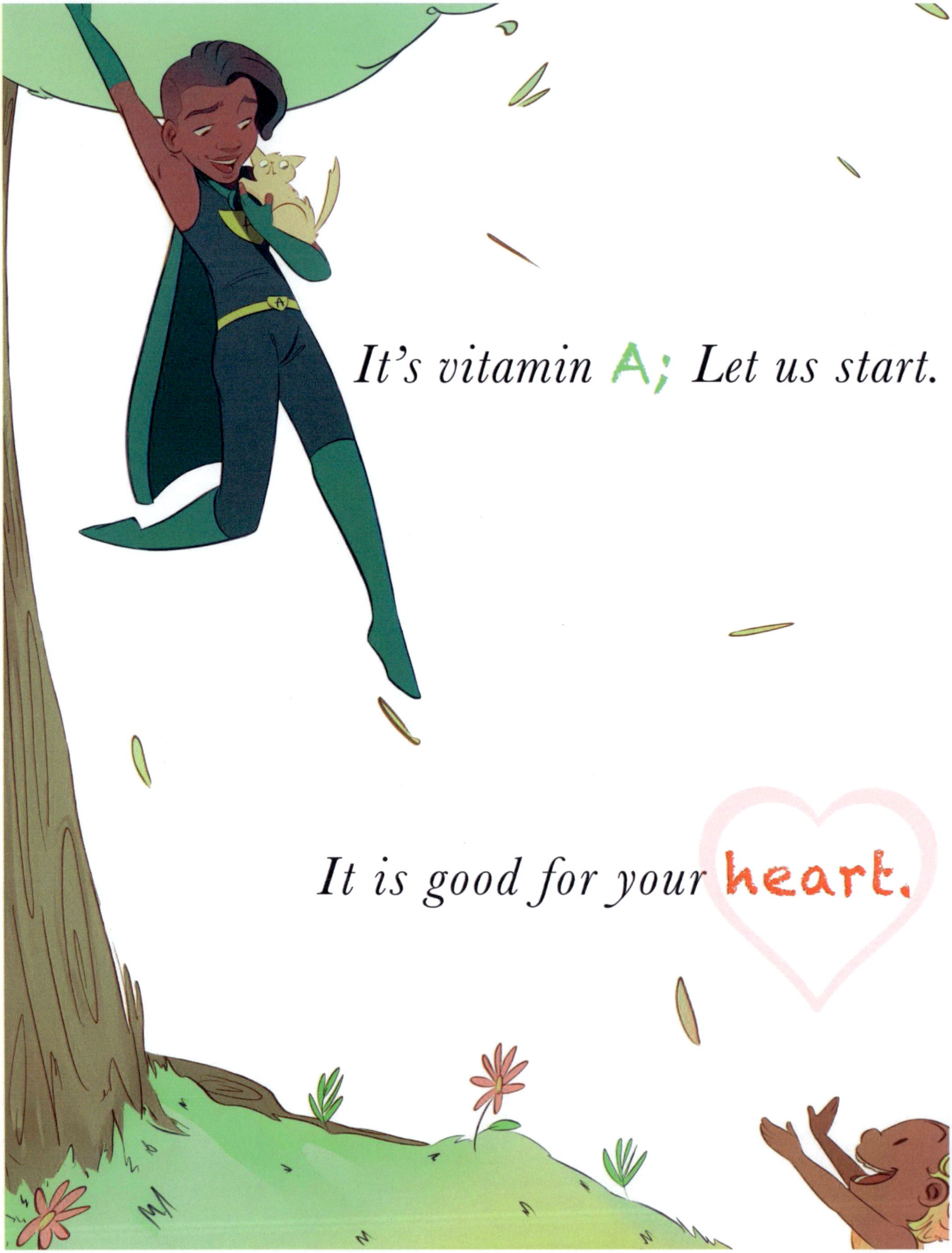

It's vitamin **A;** *Let us start.*

It is good for your **heart.**

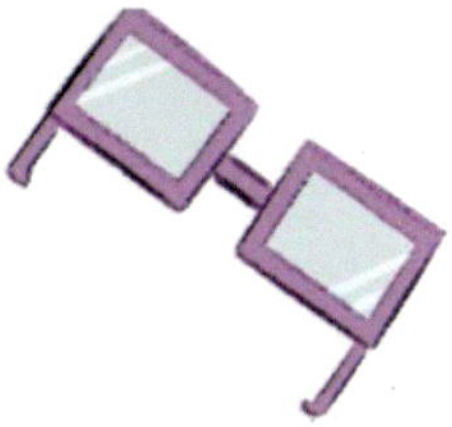

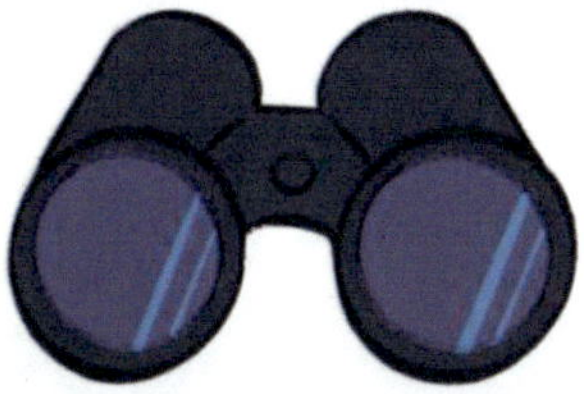

It helps you see things **close** and far

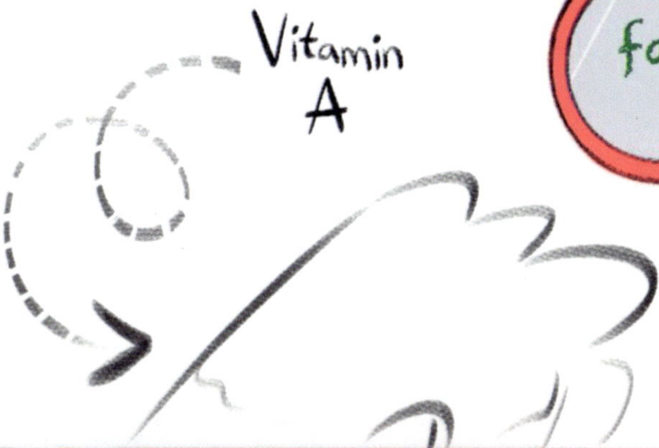

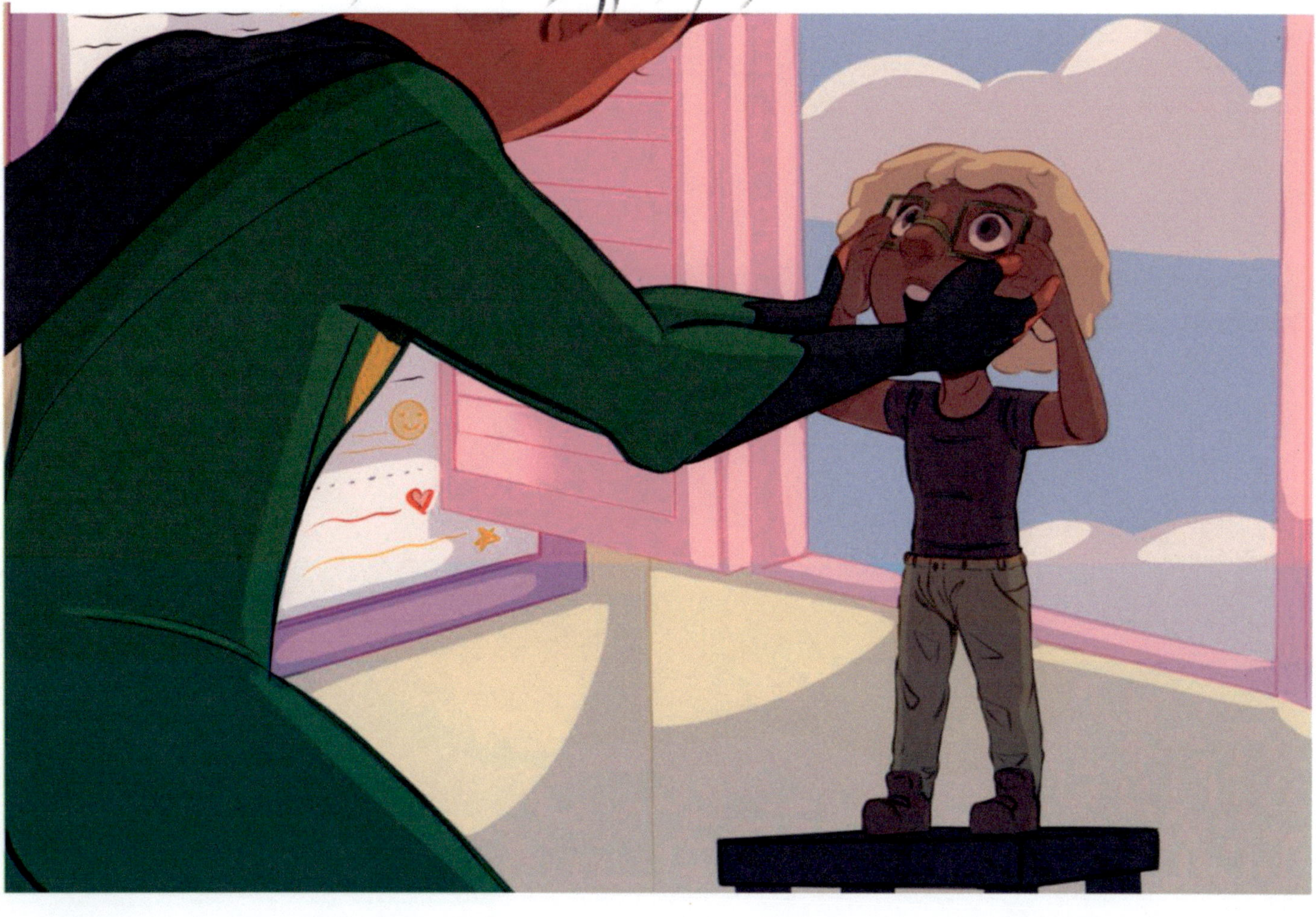

Broccoli, mangoes, tomatoes, and sweet potatoes. You can find this vitamin in all of these.

Hooray, hooray, that is Vitamin A.

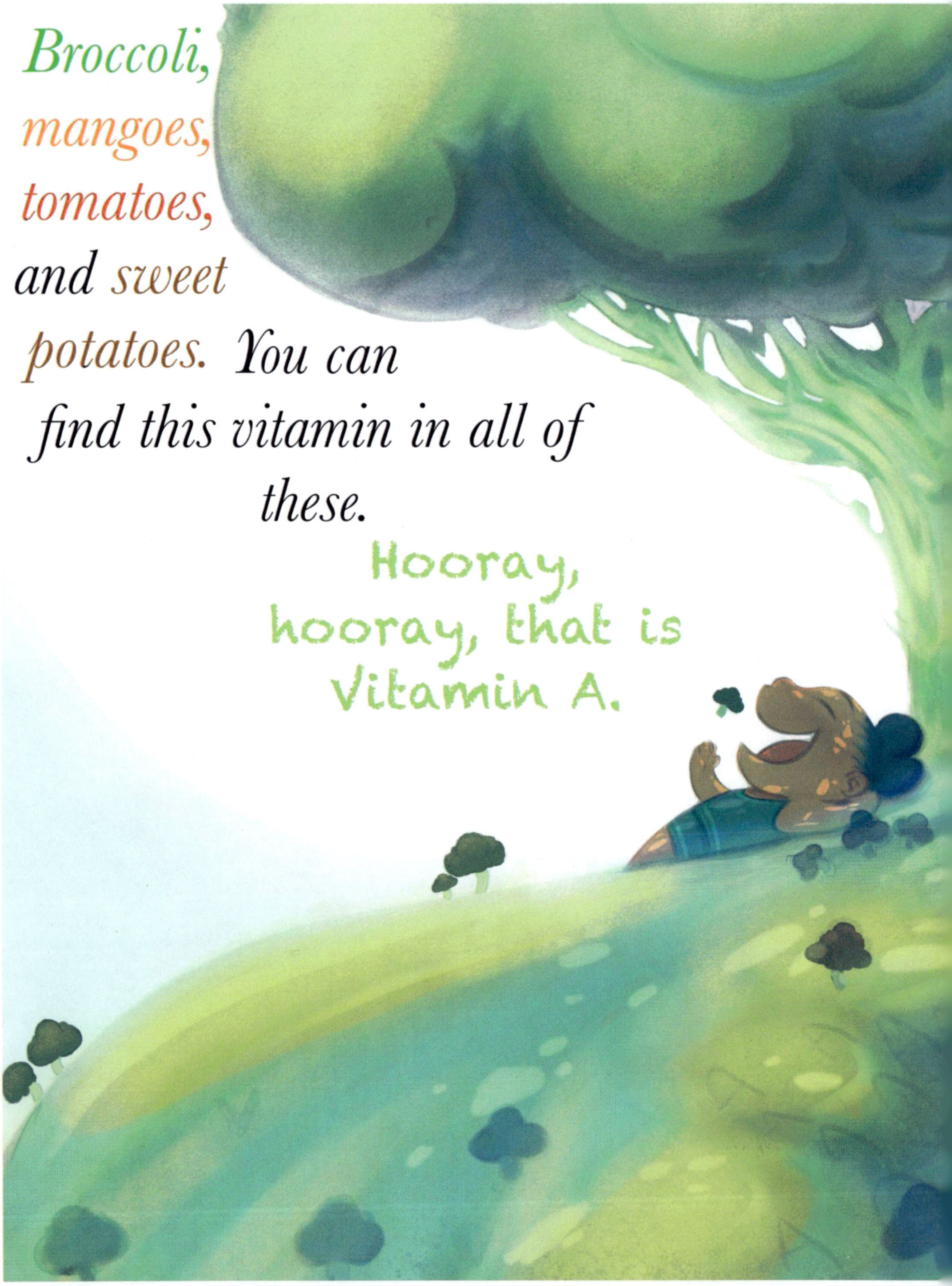

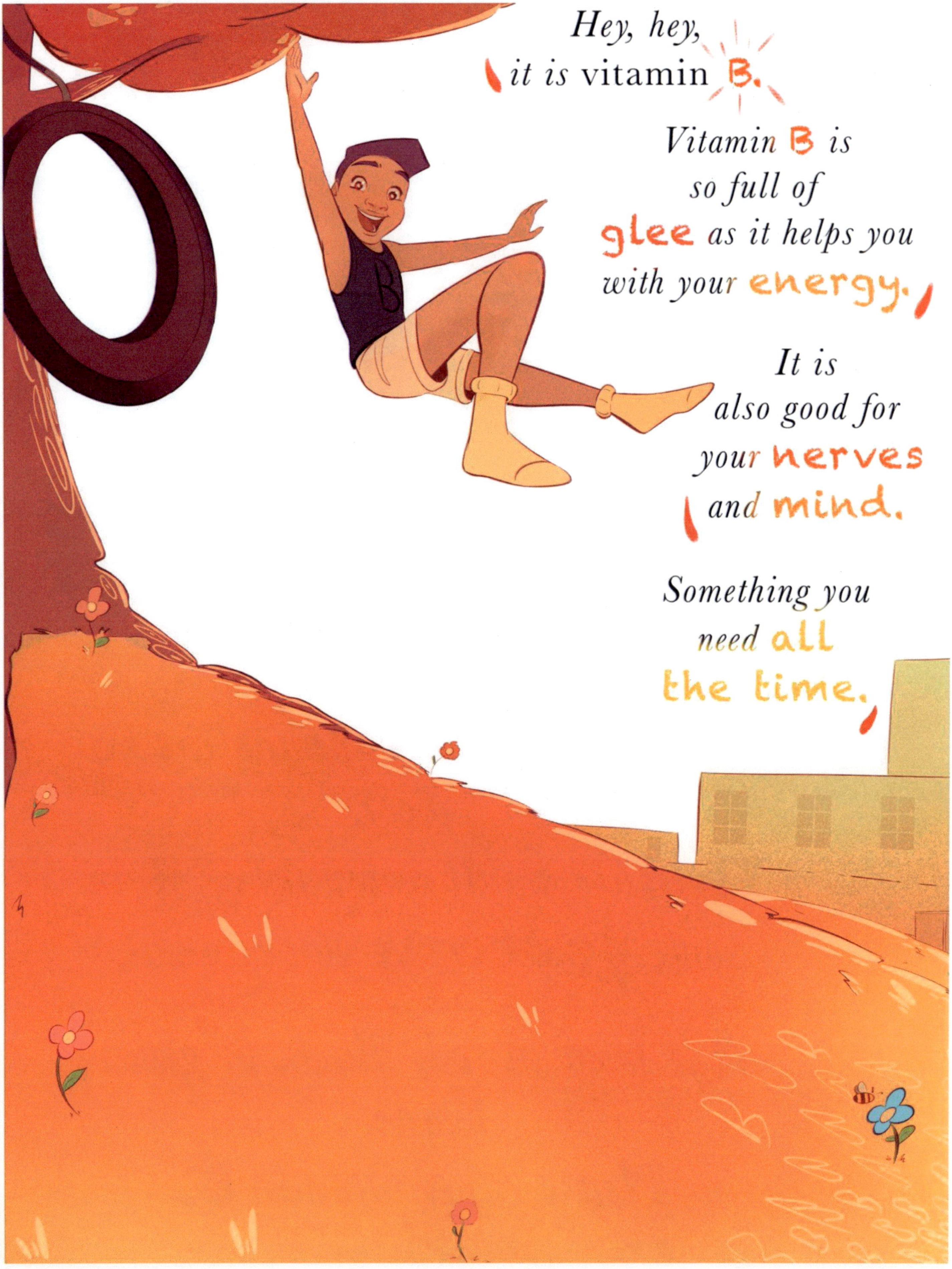

Hey, hey,
it is vitamin B.

Vitamin B *is*
so full of
glee *as it helps you*
with your energy.

It is
also good for
your nerves
and mind.

Something you
need all
the time.

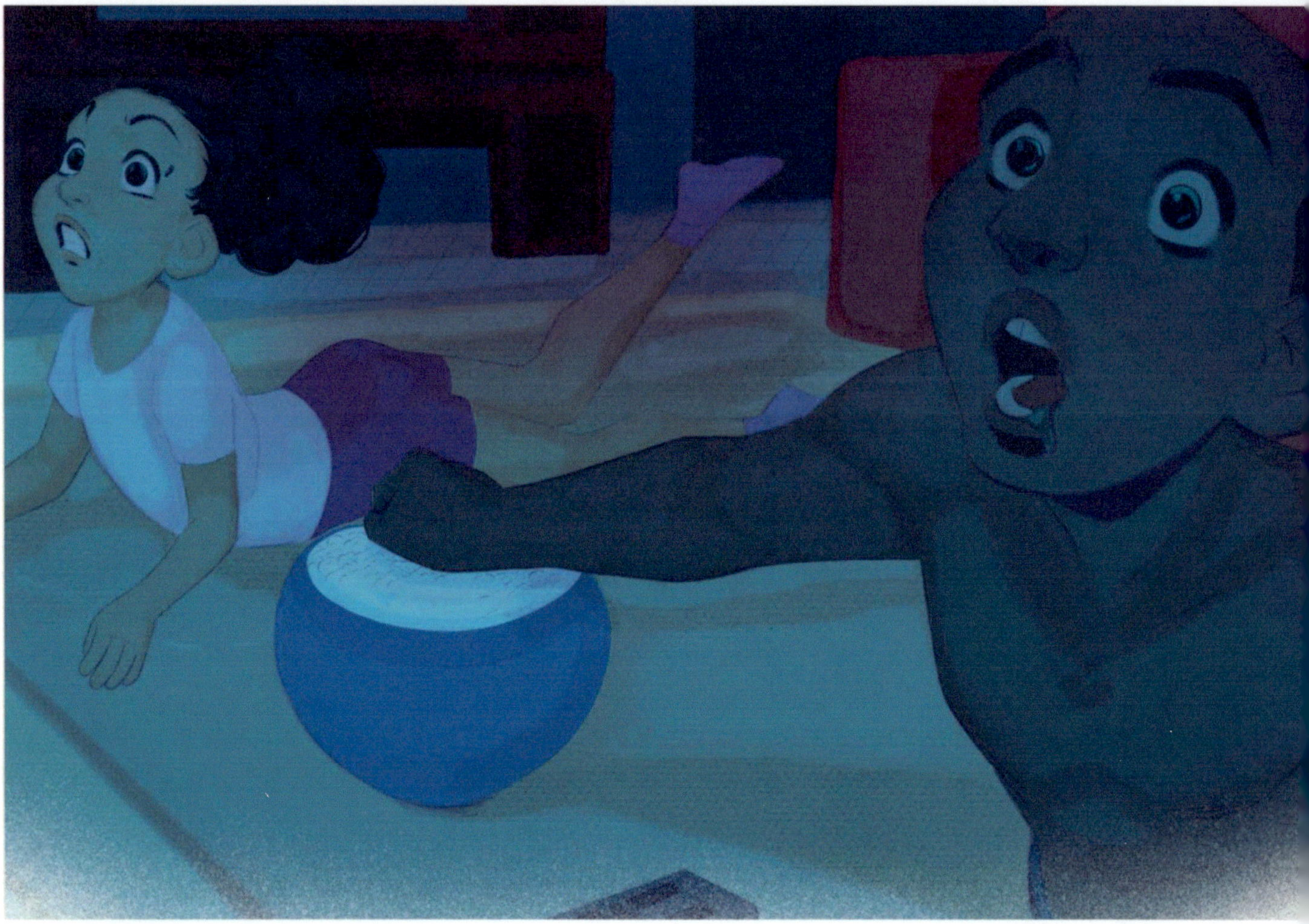

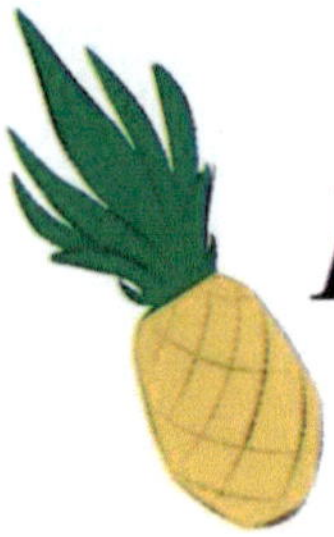

Pineapples and bananas are so *sweet.*

There are small amounts of B *in some* popcorn *you can eat.*

It is even in red, black, or green beans.

Please enjoy vitamin B.

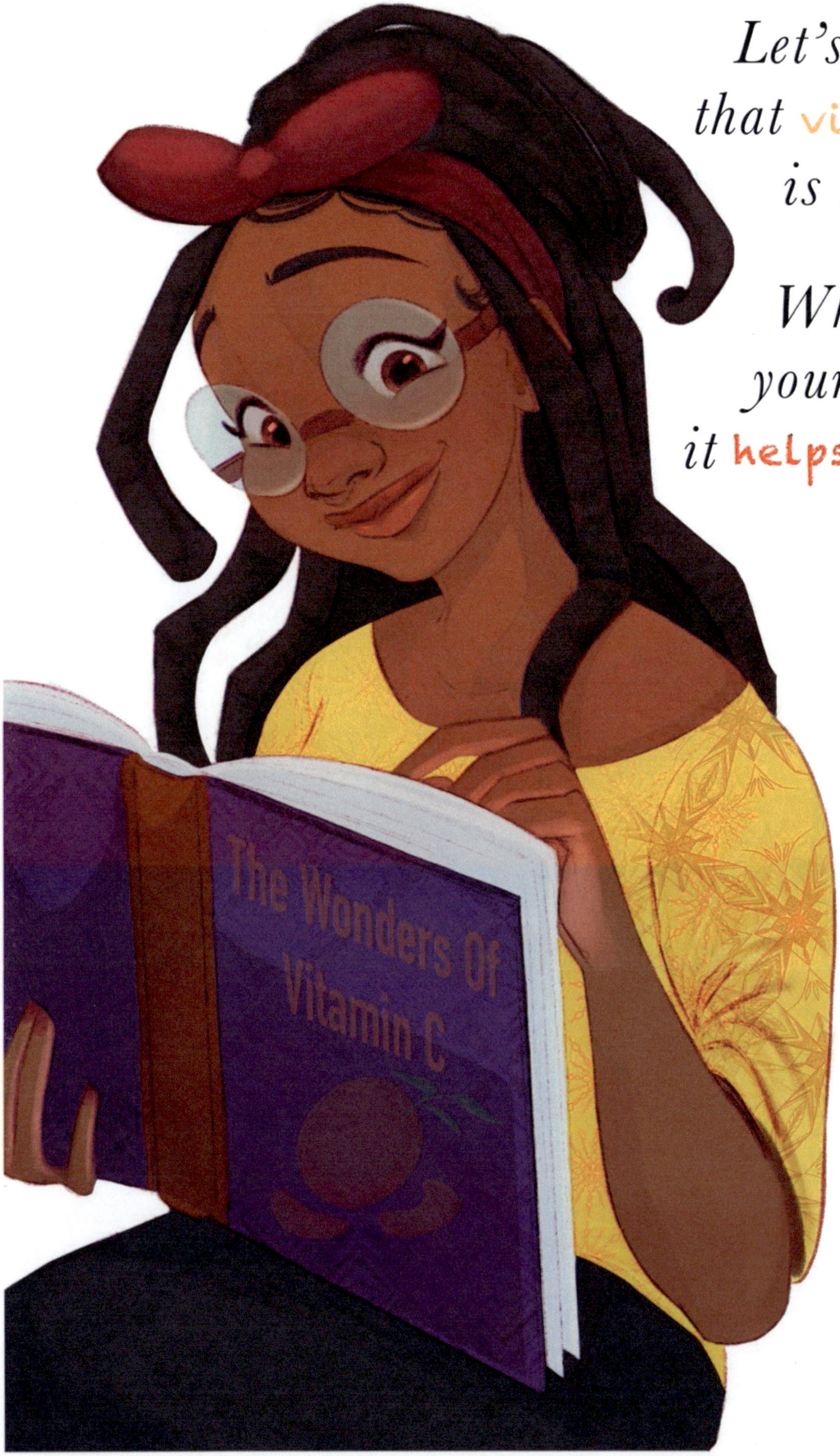

Let's cheer
that vitamin C
is here.

When in
your meal,
it helps you heal.

Its job
is to
help make
you
better
when you
are ill.

From blueberries, grapes and
strawberries. Yup, yup, yu
Even the orange juic
In your cup. It keeps yo
well and on the beat
That is the role of

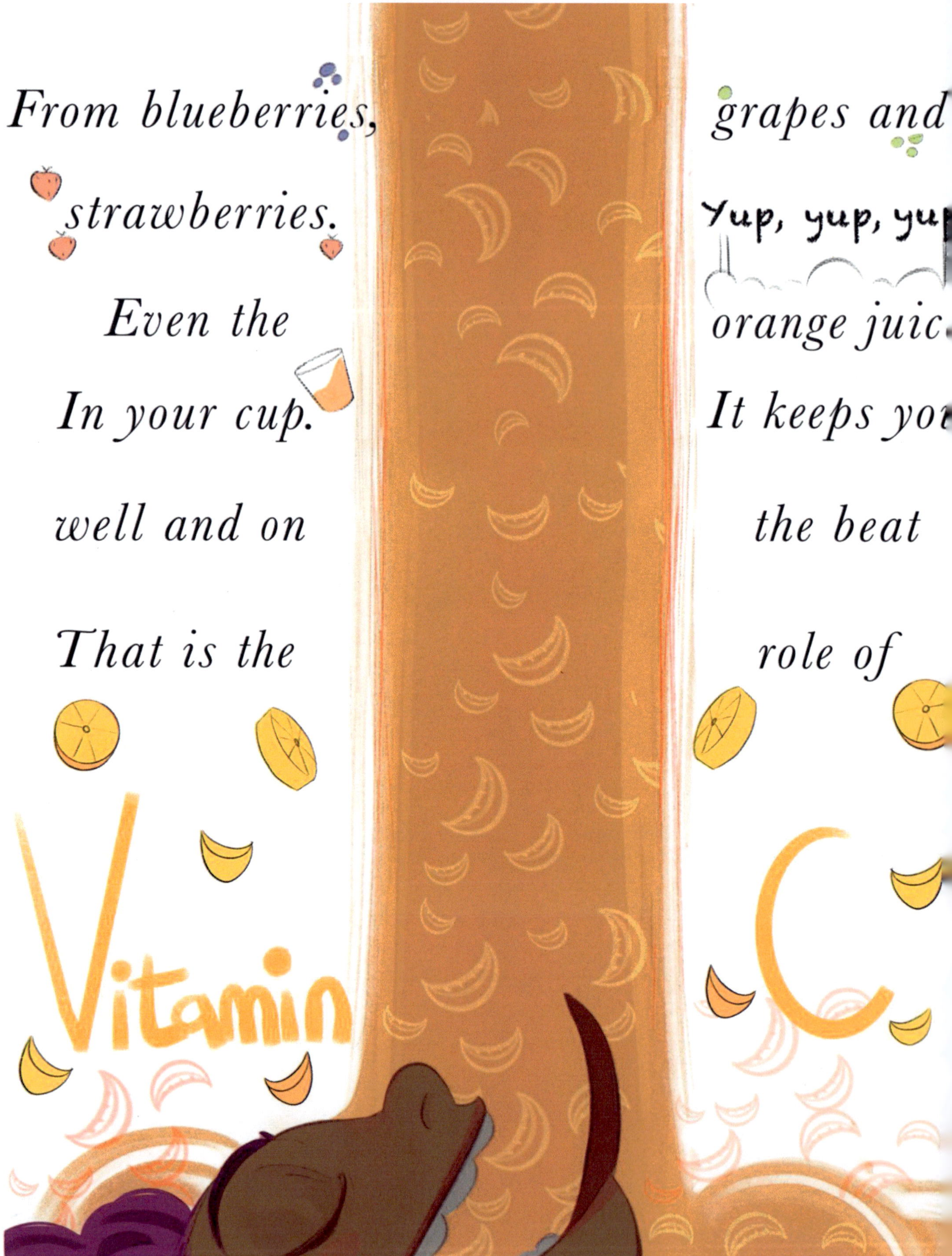

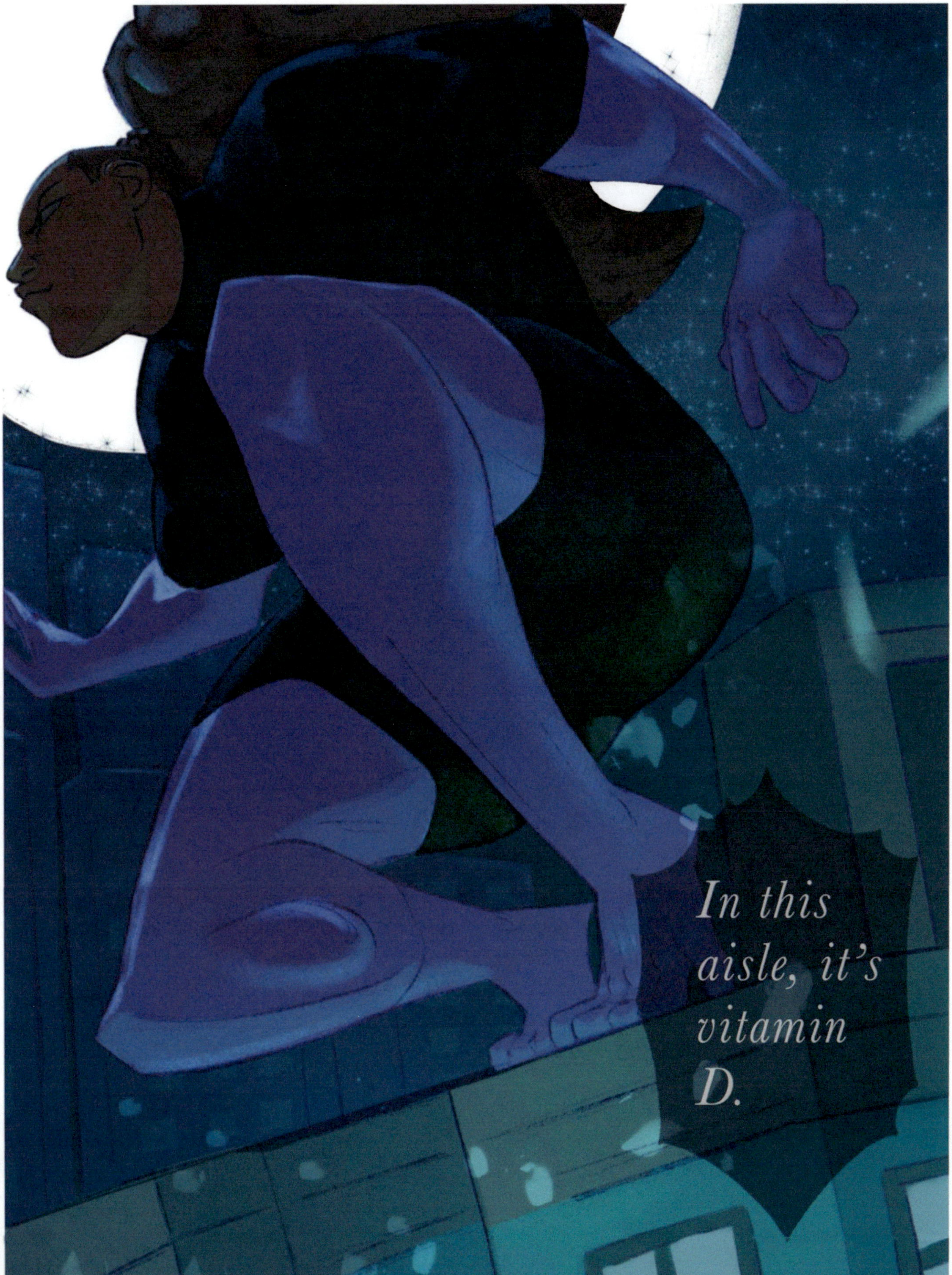
In this aisle, it's vitamin D.

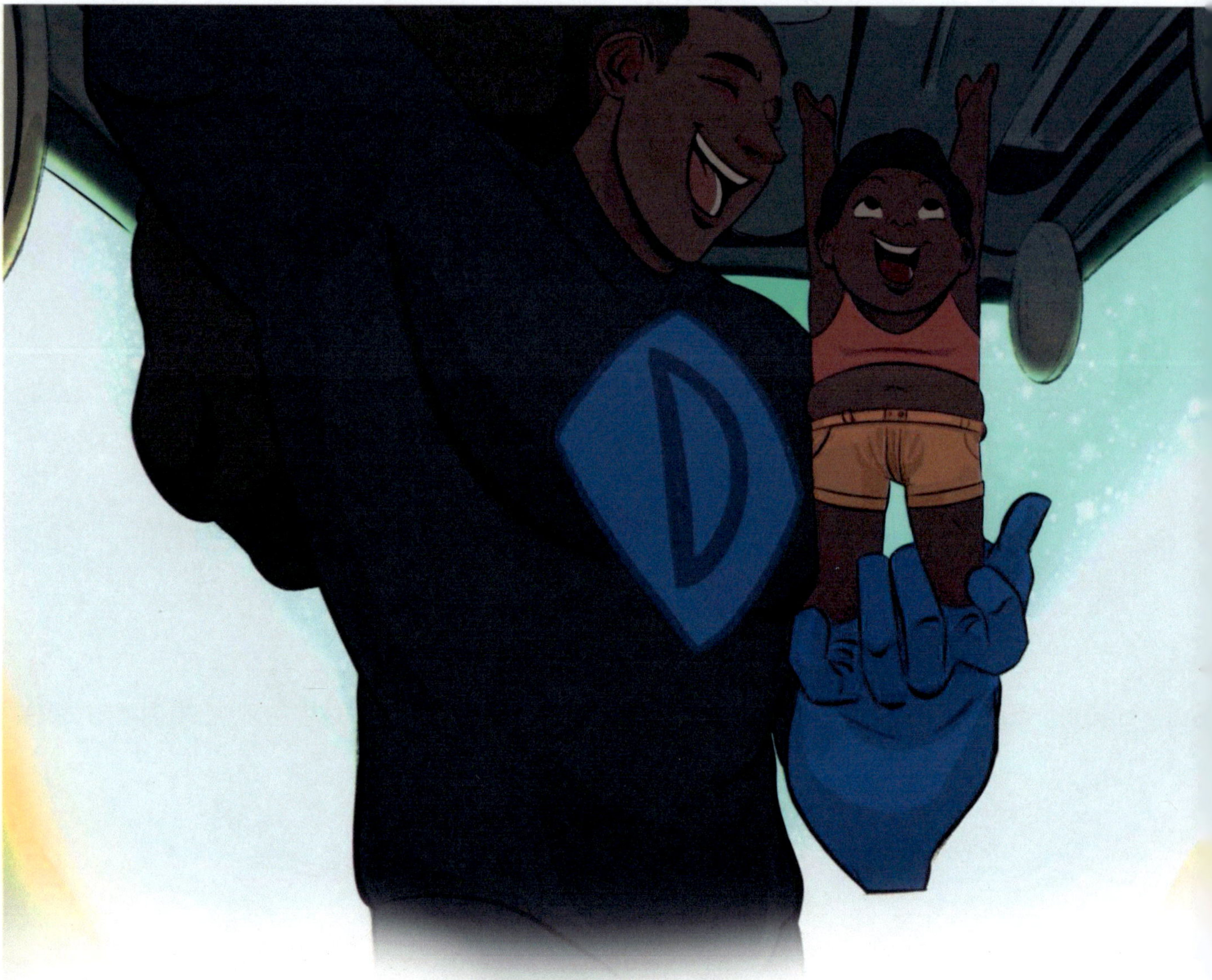

It builds strong bones and teeth for strong bites.

Be sure to get in the sun-light.

Add some mushrooms to
your savory foods.

You can eat them to
lighten your mood.

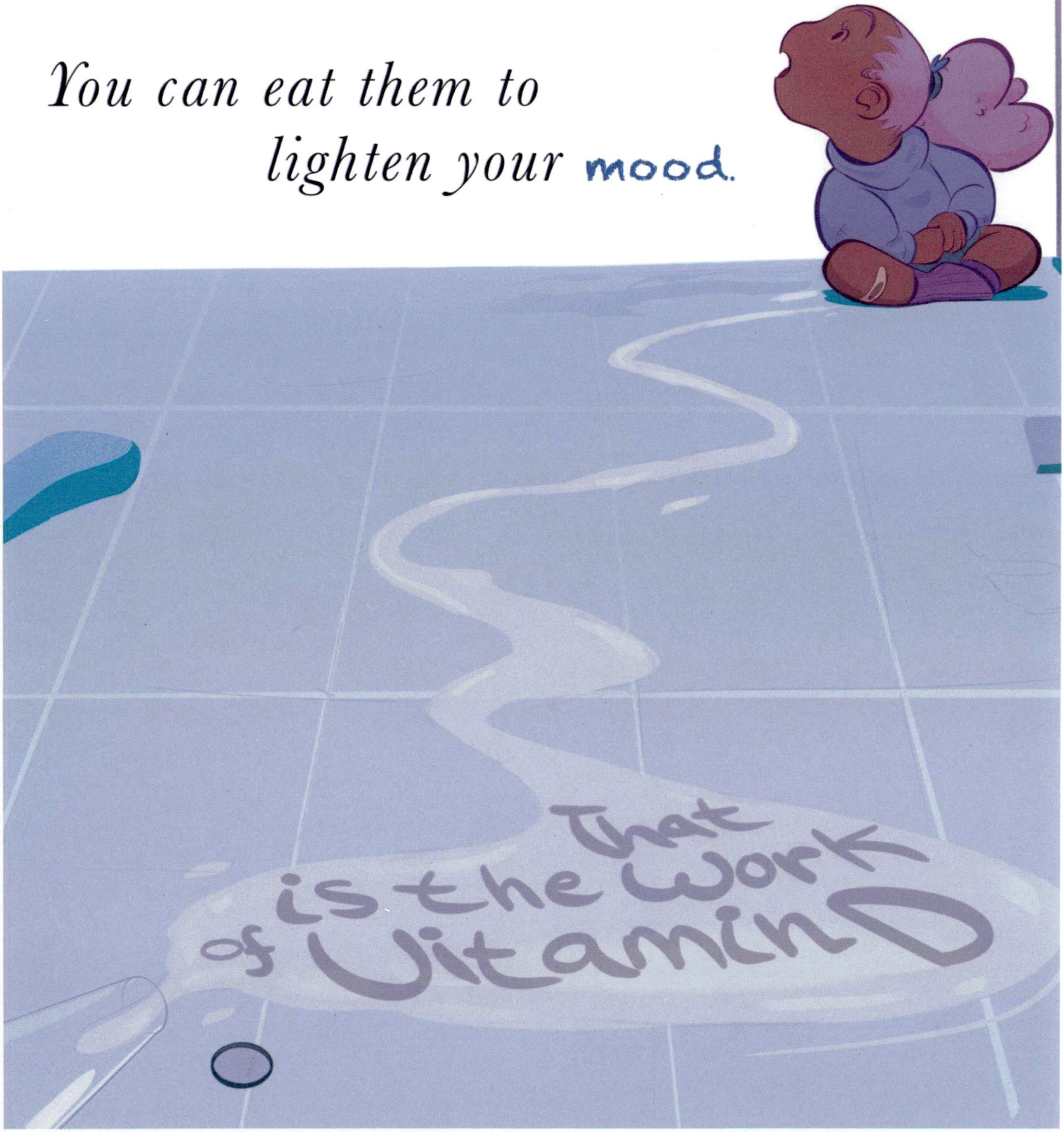

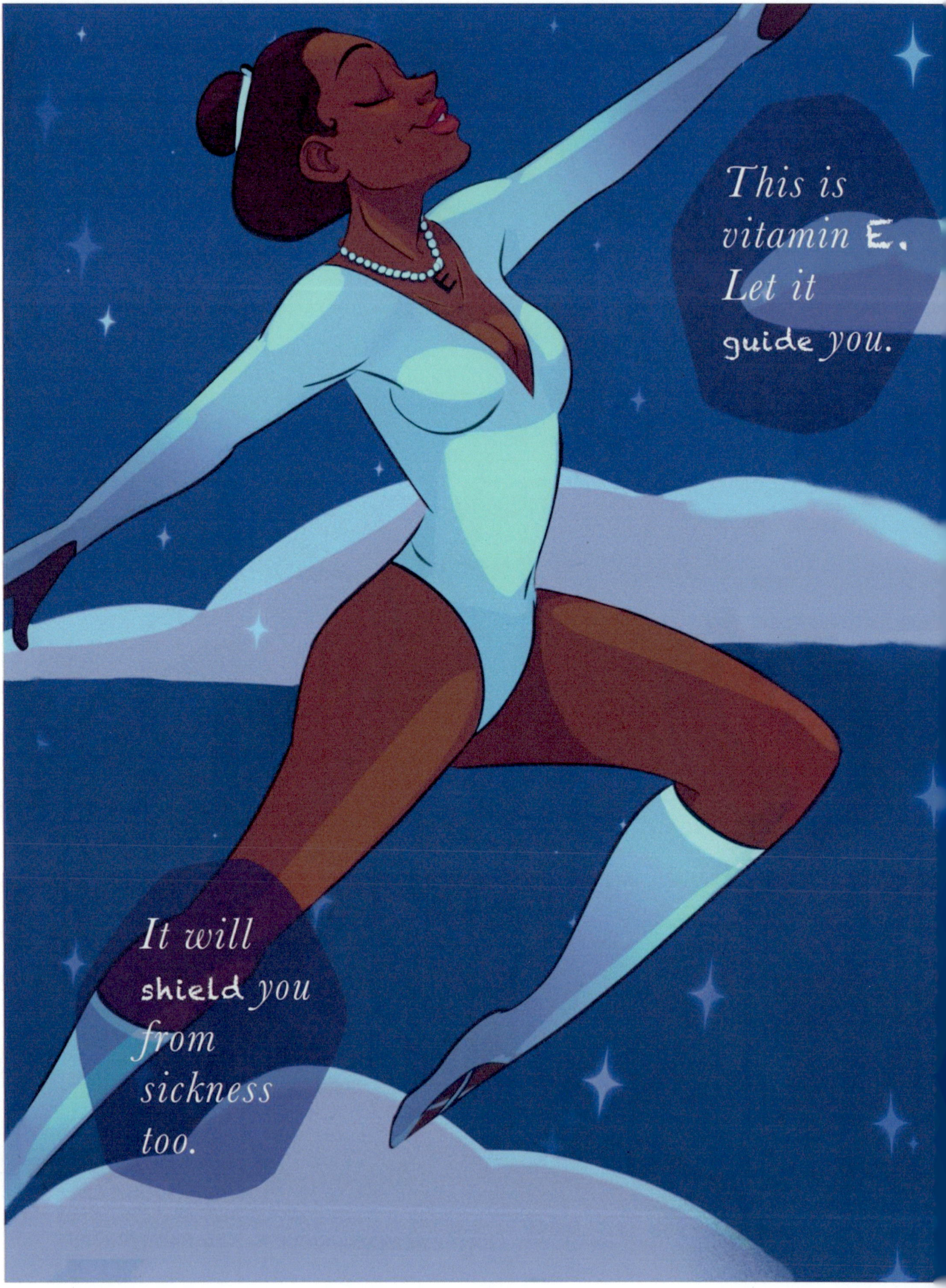
This is vitamin E. Let it guide you.
It will shield you from sickness too.

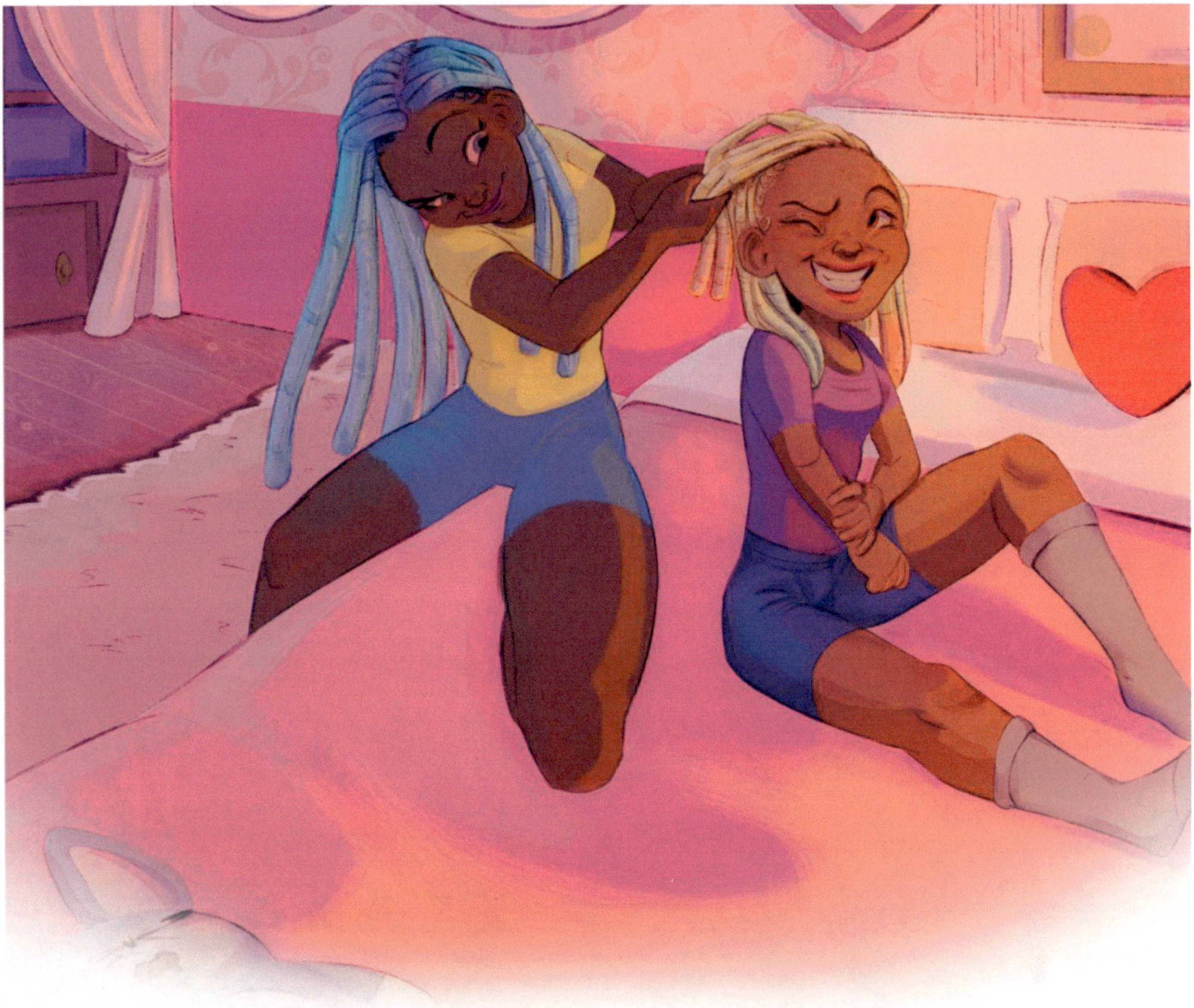

For skin and hair. So worthwhile.

With E, the only wrinkles will be from our smiles.

This is something
good to know.
That with E,
you will always glow.

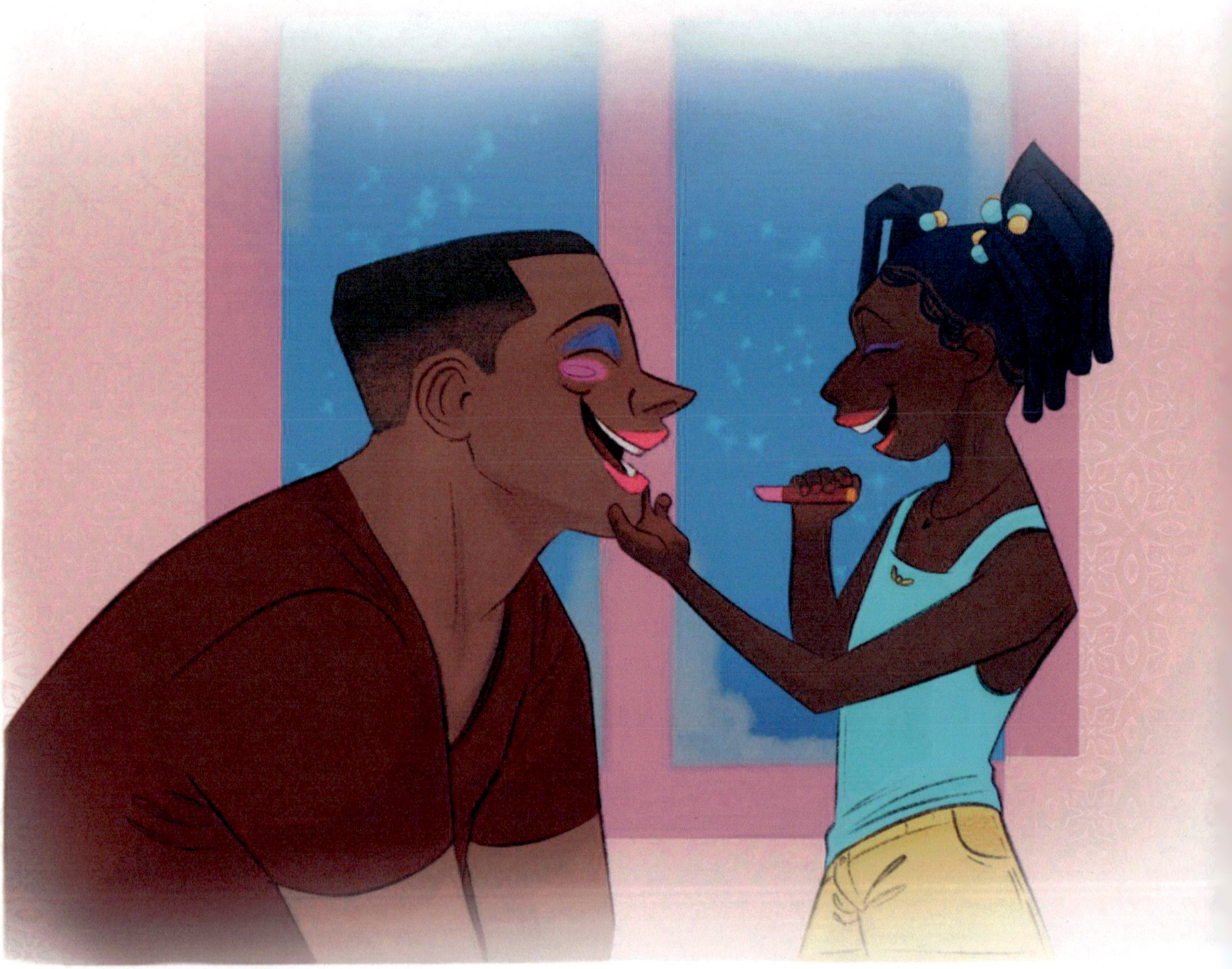

Let's snack on almonds, peanut butter, and sunflower seeds.

Vitamin E is in all of these.

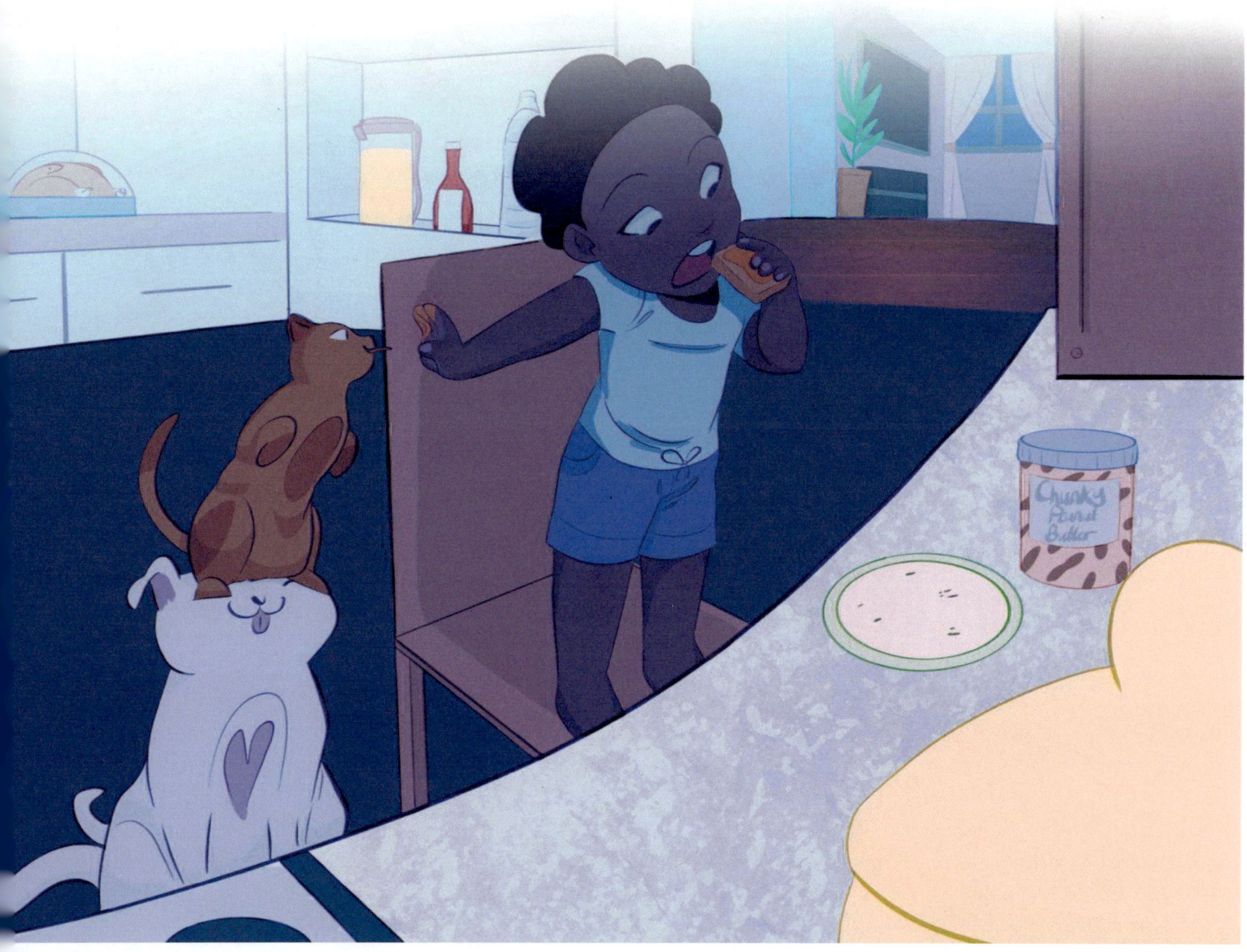

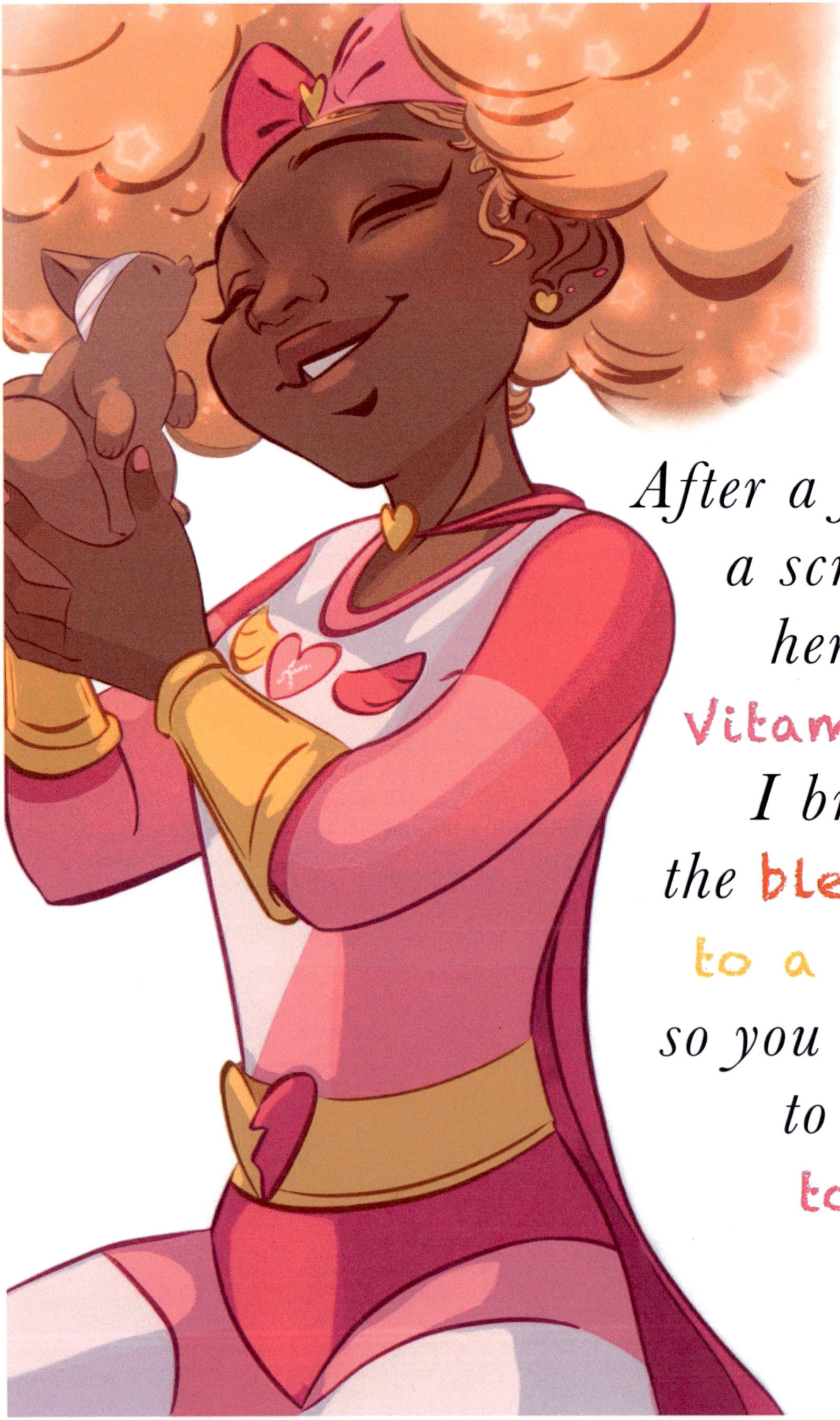

After a fall and
a scrape,
here's
Vitamin K.
I bring
the bleeding
to a stop,
so you can rise
to the
top.

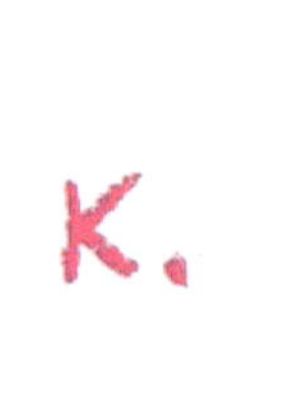

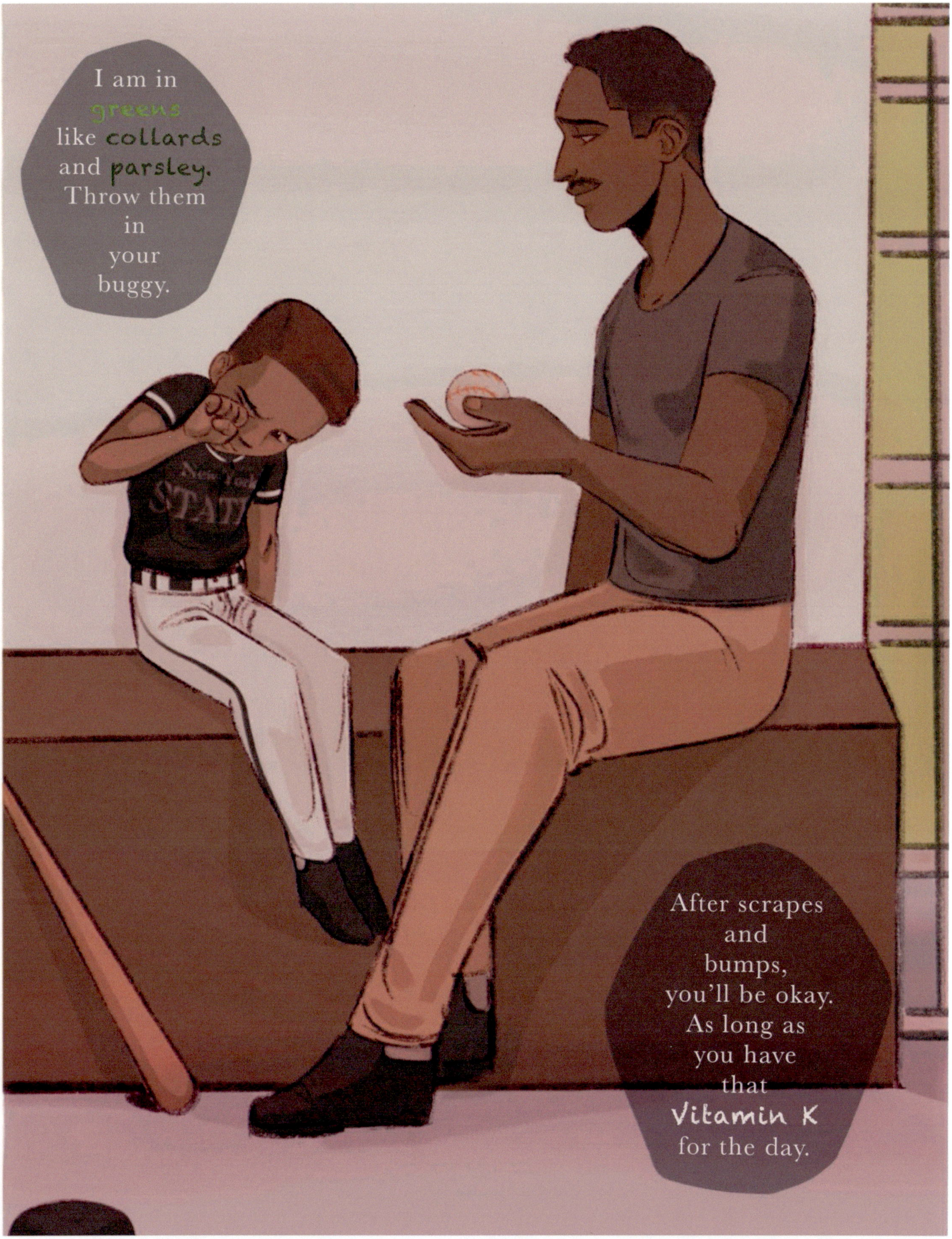
I am in greens like collards and parsley. Throw them in your buggy.
After scrapes and bumps, you'll be okay. As long as you have that Vitamin K for the day.

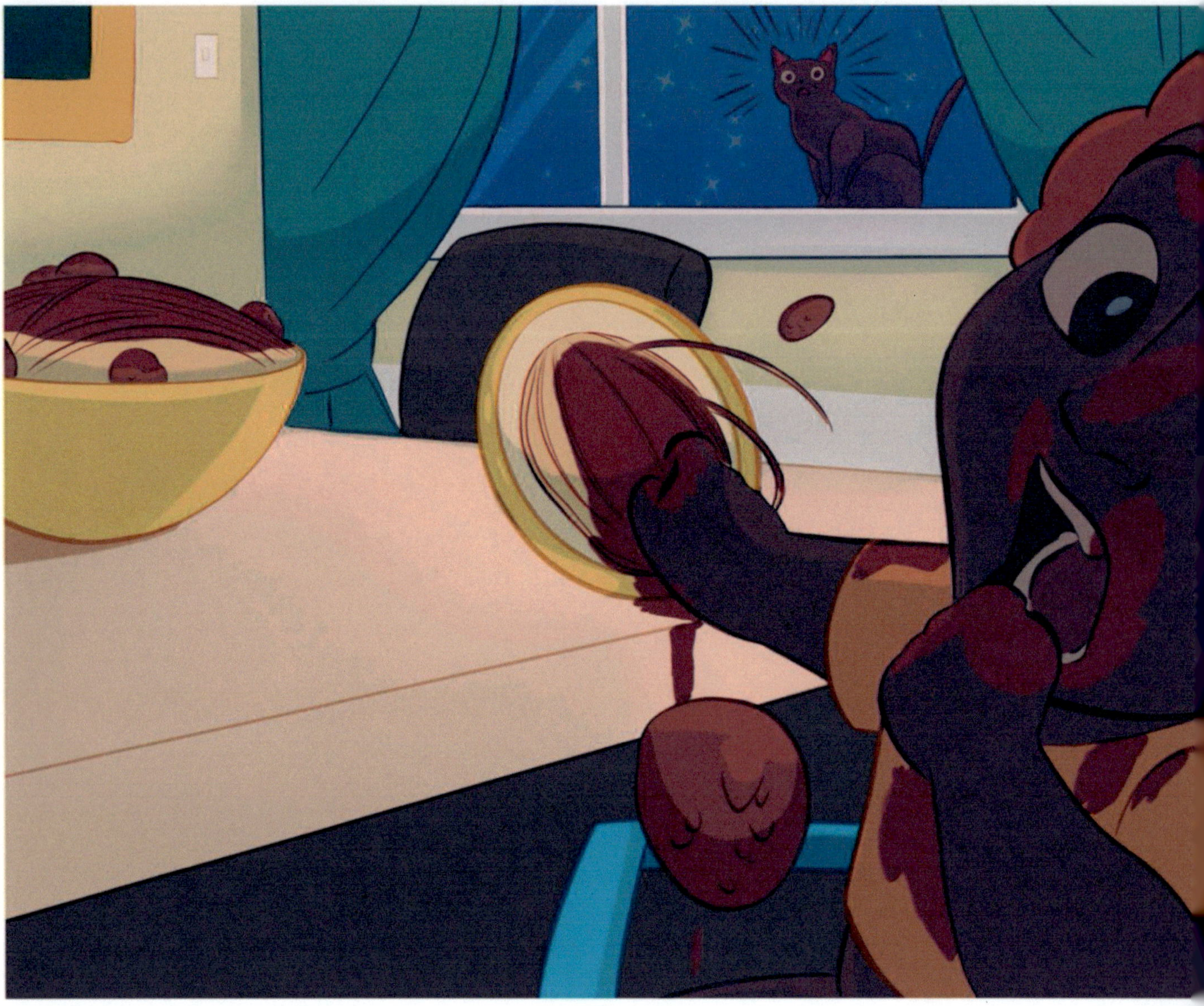

Vitamin-rich foods also keeps
your tummy full.
Many are in other fruits and veggies,
bright and colorful.

Your knowledge is now broader.
Also, remember to drink your water.

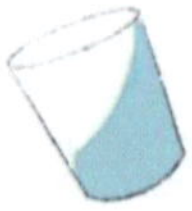

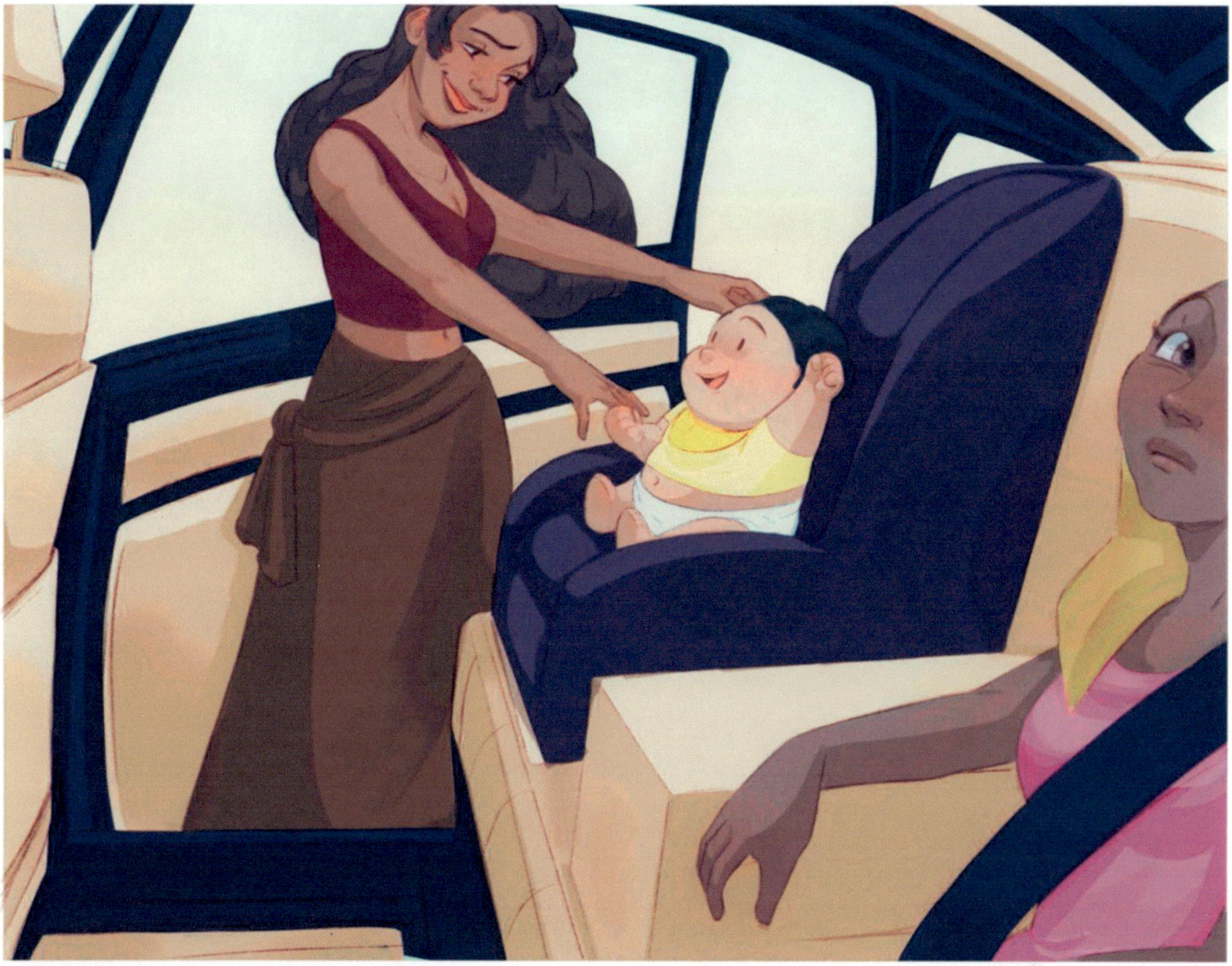

Let's go back home to eat
healthy and clean.

So you all will grow to be the most
extraordinary grown-ups
the world has ever seen.

References

- General information on child nutrition: United States Department of Agriculture. (Accessed July 2023). Children. Retrieved from https://www.nutrition.gov/topics/nutrition-life-stage/children

Vitamin A

- Vitamin A. (Revised 2021 January). Retrieved from https://ods.od.nih.gov/factsheets/VitaminA-Consumer/

- Sweet potatoes: The Nutrition Source: **Sweet potatoes** (2021) Retrieved from https://www.hsph.harvard.edu/nutritionsource/food-features/sweet-potatoes/

- Sweet potatoes: American sweet potato marketing institute (2017). Health and nutrition. Retrieved from https://americansweetpotato.org/health-nutrition/ Accessed April 7th, 2023

- Broccoli: Food Data Central. (2018). Broccoli, raw. Retrieved from https://fdc.nal.usda.gov/fdc-app.html#/food-details/170379/nutrients. Accessed April 7th, 2023

- Mangoes: National Mango Board (2023). Mango Nutrition. Retrieved from. https://www.mango.org/mango-nutrition/#:~:text=Mangos%20contain%20over%2020%20different,of%20your%20daily%20vitamin%20B6. Accessed April 7th, 2023.

- Tomatoes: Swartzendruber, K. (2018). Tomatoes provide many health benefits. Retrieved From https://www.canr.msu.edu/news/tomatoes_provide_many_health_benefits#:~:text=One%20serving%20of%20tomatoes%20provides,of%20the%20daily%20recommended%20amount. Accessed April 7th, 2023.

Vitamin B

- The Nutrition Source: B vitamins. (2021). Retrieved from https://www.hsph.harvard.edu/nutritionsource/vitamins/vitamin-b/

- Pineapple: Ivanova NN, Khomich LM, Perova IB, Eller KI. [Pineapple juice nutritional profile]. Vopr Pitan. 2019;88(2):73-82. Russian. doi: 10.24411/0042-8833-2019-10020. Epub 2019 Mar 13. PMID: 31233691.

- Pineapple: Pineapple composition and nutrition. Ancos, B., Sánchez-Moreno, C., González-Aguilar, G. (2016). Functional properties of pineapple. Retrieved from https://doi.org/10.1002/9781118967355.ch13. Accessed Apr 7, 2023.

- **Bananas**: László Sági , Gregory D. May , Serge Remy & Rony Swennen (1998). Recent Developments in Biotechnological Research on Bananas (Musa spp.), Biotechnology and Genetic Engineering Reviews, 15:1, 313-328, DOI: 10.1080/02648725.1998.10647960

- **Popcorn**: McDonnell, K. (2017). Popcorn nutrition facts: A healthy, low-calorie snack? Retrieved from: https://www.healthline.com/nutrition/popcorn-nutrition-and-health

- **Red Beans**: Bhatty R.S. Composition and Quality of Lentil (Lens-culinaris Medik)—A review. Food Sci. Technol. Int. 1988;21:144–160. doi: 10.1016/S0315-5463(88)70770-1.

- **Green Beans**: Williamson, L. (2022). Green beans can be one of the healthiest dishes at the holiday table. Retrieved from: https://www.heart.org/en/news/2022/11/22/green-beans-can-be-one-of-the-healthiest-dishes-at-the-holiday-table#:~:text=Not%20only%20are%20they%20relatively,which%20helps%20regulate%20blood%20pressure.

- **Black Beans**: US Department of Agriculture. (2018). Beans, black, mature seeds, cooked, boiled, with salt. https://fdc.nal.usda.gov/fdc-app.html#/food-details/175237/nutrients

Vitamin C

- Vitamin C. (Updated 2021 March). Retrieved from https://ods.od.nih.gov/factsheets/VitaminC-Consumer/

- Nutrition ranking tool. (Accessed 2021) Retrieved from https://tools.myfooddata.com/nutrient-ranking-tool/Vitamin-C/Fruits/Highest/Household/Simple/No

- Grapes: Cleveland Clinic (2021). 10 Health Benefits of Grapes. Retrieved from https://health.clevelandclinic.org/health-benefits-of-grapes/

- Strawberries, blueberries, oranges. Top 10 Foods Highest in Vitamin C (2021). Retrieved from https://www.myfooddata.com/articles/vitamin-c-foods.php

- Blueberries: Wergin, A. (2022). The power of **blueberries**. Retrieved from https://www.mayoclinichealthsystem.org/hometown-health/speaking-of-health/the-power-of-blueberries#:~:text=A%20one%2Dcup%20serving%20of,means%20they%20contain%20mostly%20water.

Vitamin D

- Vitamin D. (Revised 2021 March). Retrieved from https://ods.od.nih.gov/factsheets/VitaminD-Consumer/
- 7 Healthy foods that are high in vitamin D (Accessed 2021 March) https://www.healthline.com/nutrition/9-foods-high-in-vitamin-d#Vitamin-D-and-calcium
- Mushrooms: D.B.Haytowitz. Vitamin D in Mushrooms Retrieved from https://www.ars.usda.gov/ARSUserFiles/80400525/Articles/AICR09_Mushroom_VitD.pdf
- Mushrooms: Horst, R. (2009). Personal Communications. Heartland Assays, Inc. Ames, IA. Pehrsson PR, Haytowitz DB,

- Mushrooms: Holden JM. (2003). The USDA's National Food and Nutrient Analysis Program: Update 2002. J Food Comp Anal 16:331-341.

- Mushrooms: Roberts, J.S., Teichert, A., and McHugh, T.H. (2008). Vitamin D2 formation from postharvest UV-B treatment of mushrooms (Agaricus bisporus) and retention during storage. J. Agric. Food Chem. 56:4541-4544

- Sunlight: Ashley, R. (2018). Ask the Doctors - How much sunshine do I need for enough vitamin D? Retrieved from https://www.uclahealth.org/news/ask-the-doctors-round-sun-exposure-vital-to-vitamin-d-production#:~:text=In%20the%20winter%2C%20only%2010,sufficient%20amount%20of%20vitamin%20D. Accessed Apr 7, 2023

Vitamin E

- Vitamin E. (Revised 2021 March).Retrieved from https://ods.od.nih.gov/factsheets/VitaminE-Consumer/

- Peanut Butter: Bauer, J. The healthy perks of peanut butter. Retrieved from: https://www.denverhealthmedicalplan.org/blog/healthy-perks-peanut-butter

- Peanut Butter: Frey, M (2022) Peanut butter nutrition facts and health benefits. Retrieved from: https://www.verywellfit.com/is-peanut-butter-good-for-you-3495231?utm_term=bouncex4&utm_campaign=health_tod&utm_medium=email&utm_content=7385812&utm_source=cn_nl

- **Almonds**: Harvard T.H. Chan (2023). The nutrition Source: Vitamin E. Retrieved from: https://www.hsph.harvard.edu/nutritionsource/vitamin-e/

- **Sunflower Seeds**: Holliday, R, and Phillips, K. (2001). Health benefits of the sunflower kernel. Cereal Foods World, 46:205.

Vitamin K

- Vitamin K. (2020 February). Retrieved from https://ods.od.nih.gov/factsheets/VitaminK-Consum

- 20 Vitamin K foods that should be part of your diet. (Accessed March 2021) Retrieved from https://medalerthelp.org/blog/vitamin-k-foods/

- Collards: University of Iowa Hospital and Clinics. (2021). Warfarin, your diet, and vitamin K foods https://uihc.org/educational-resources/warfarin-your-diet-and-vitamin-k-foods#:~:text=The%20most%20common%20foods%20with,spinach%2C%20cabbage%2C%20and%20lettuce.

- Parsley: University of Rochester Medical Center. (2023). Nutrition facts; parsley, raw, 1 cup.

Bonus Material 1

These are actual photos of the food items in the rhyme.

VITAMIN A

Sweet Potato (Baked)

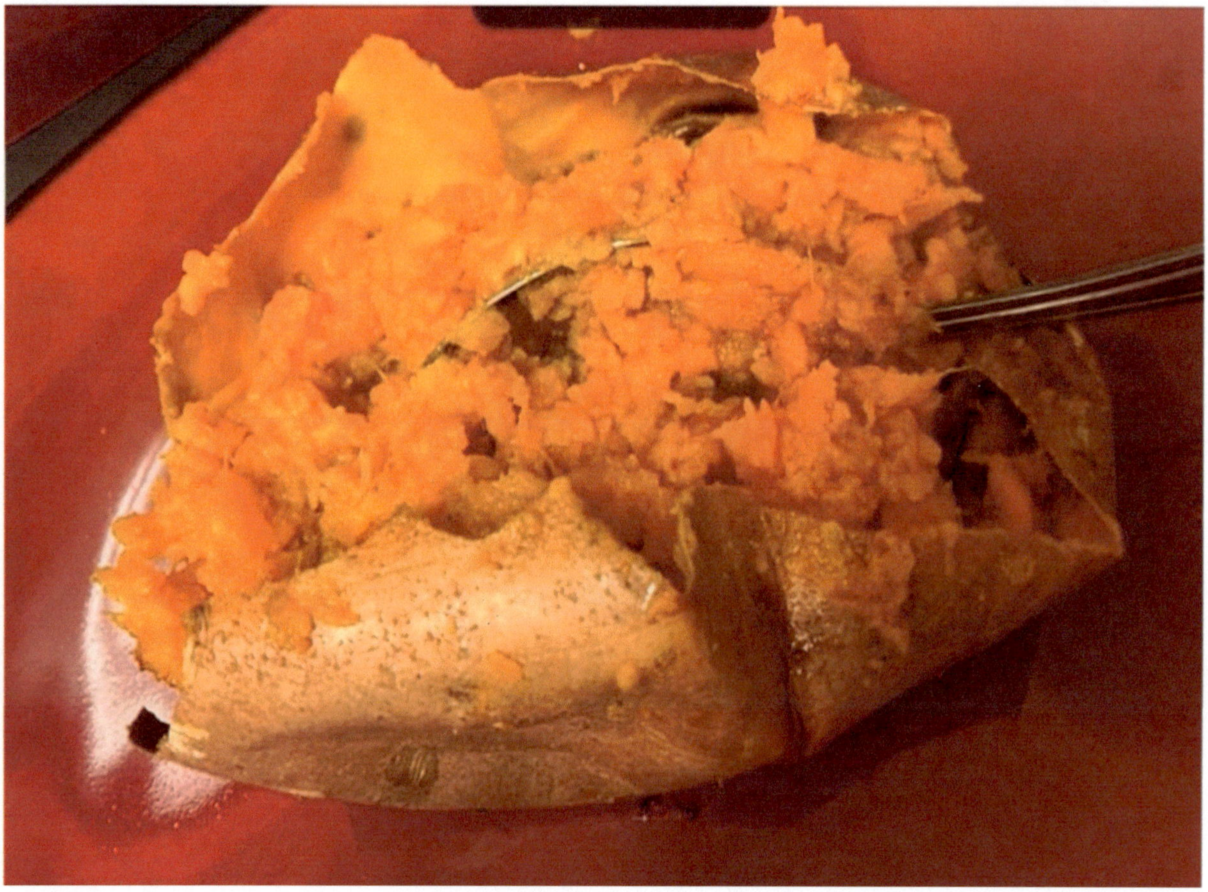

Sweet Potatoes (peeled, sliced, and raw)

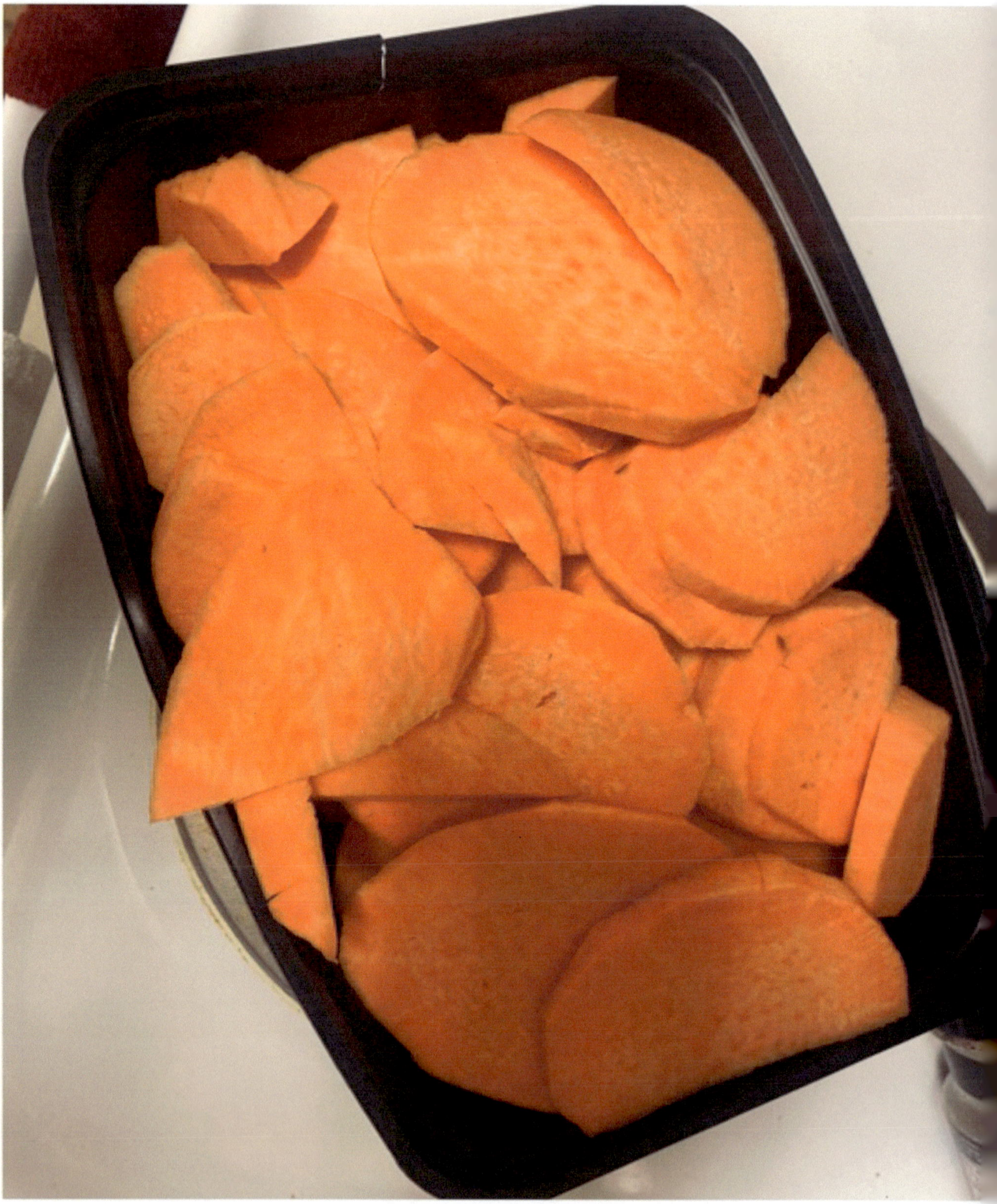

Broccoli

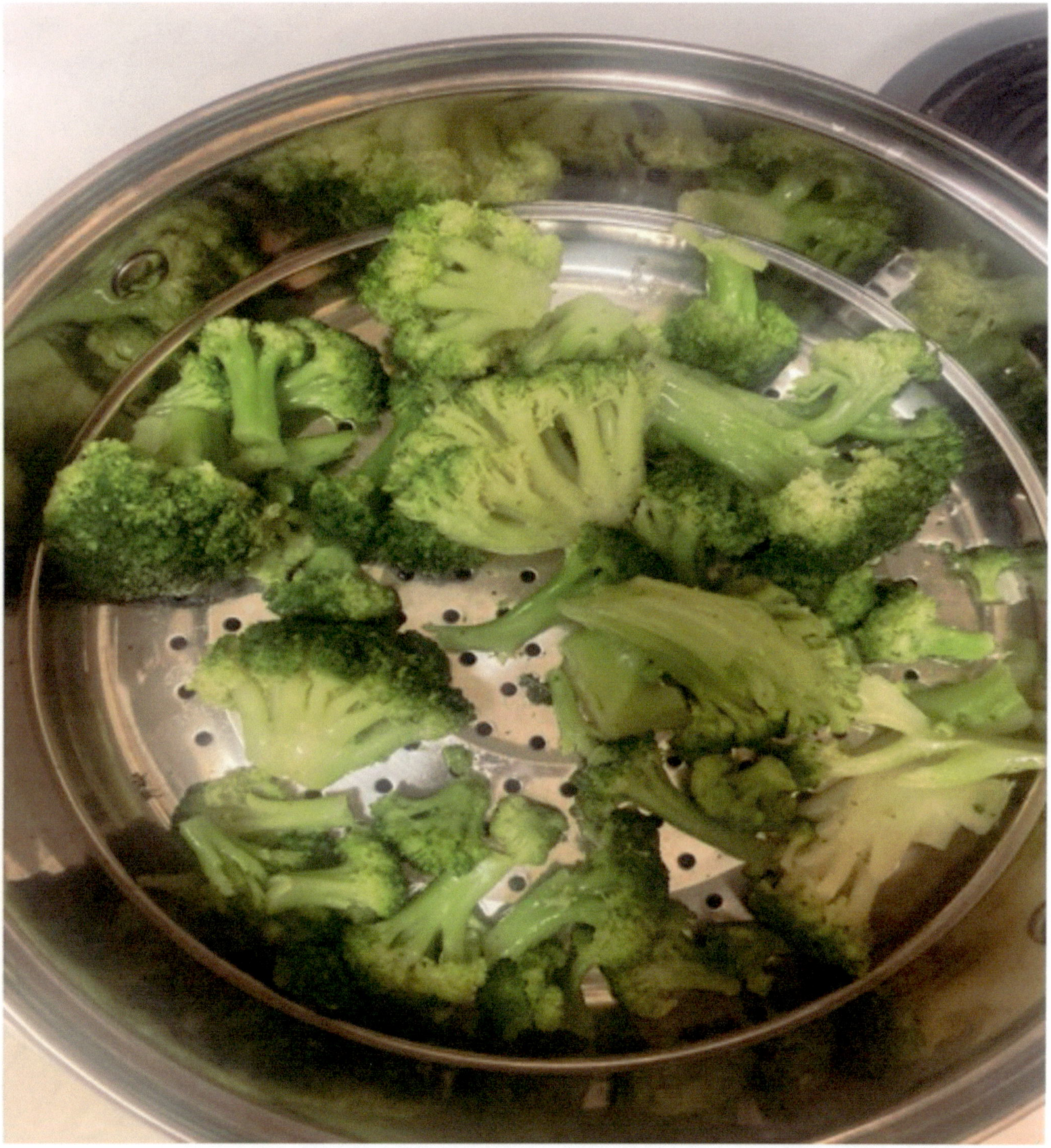

Mango

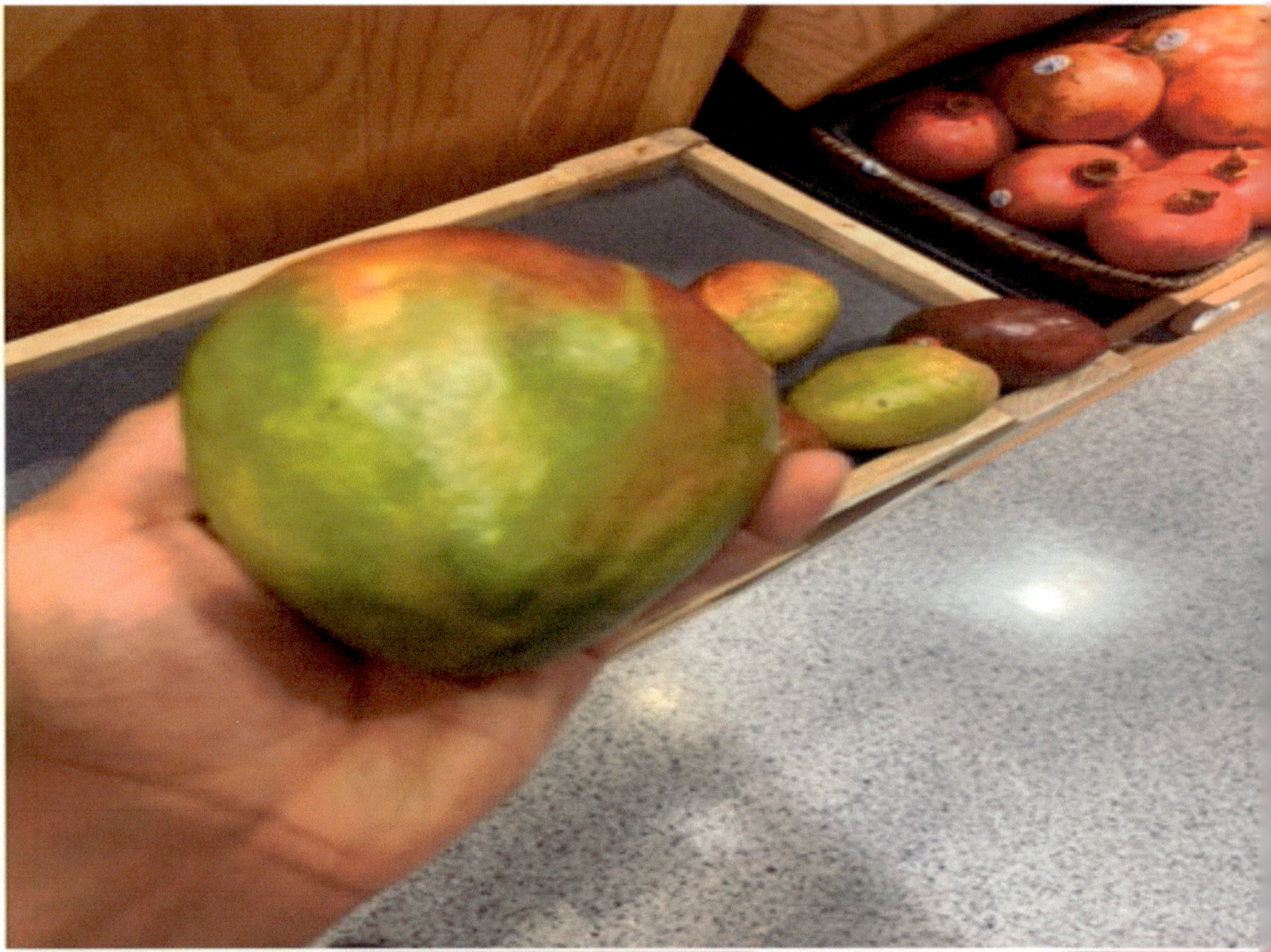

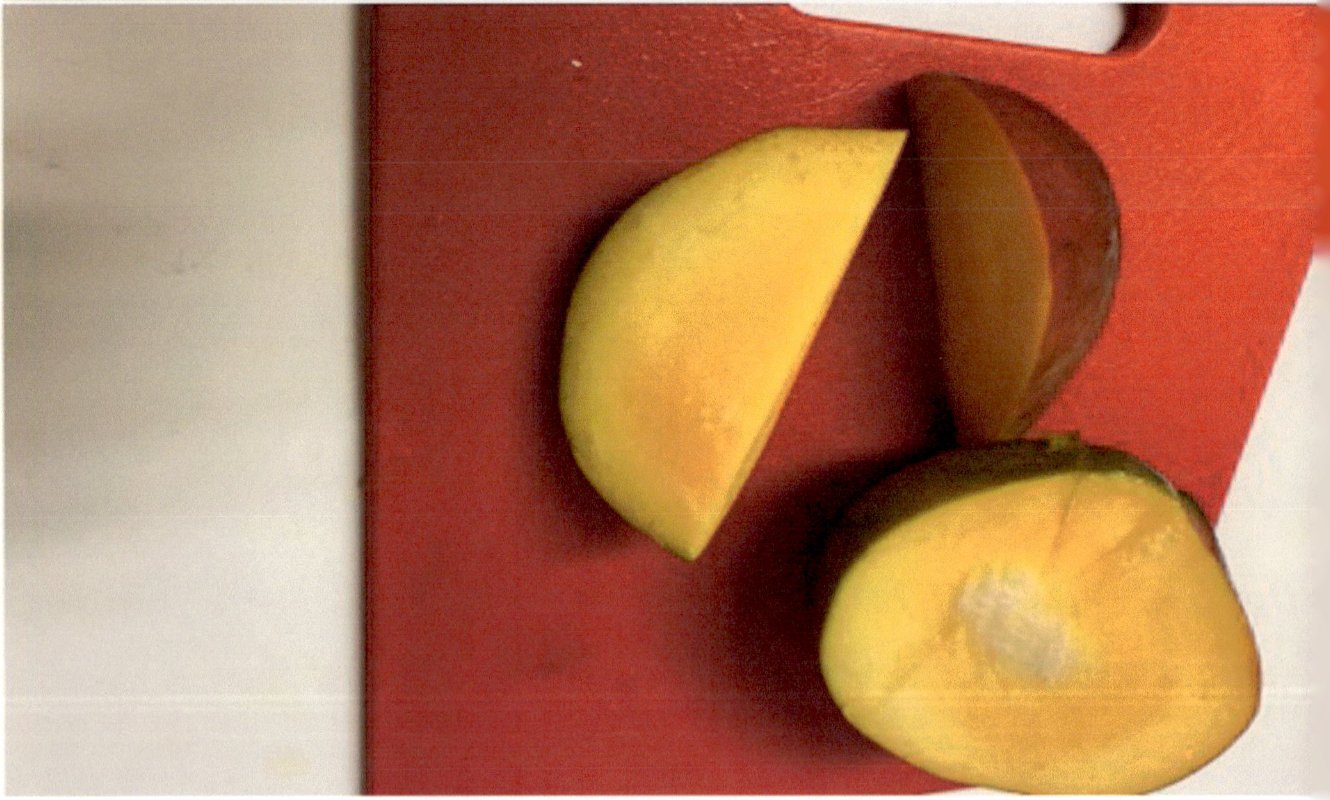

Tomatoes

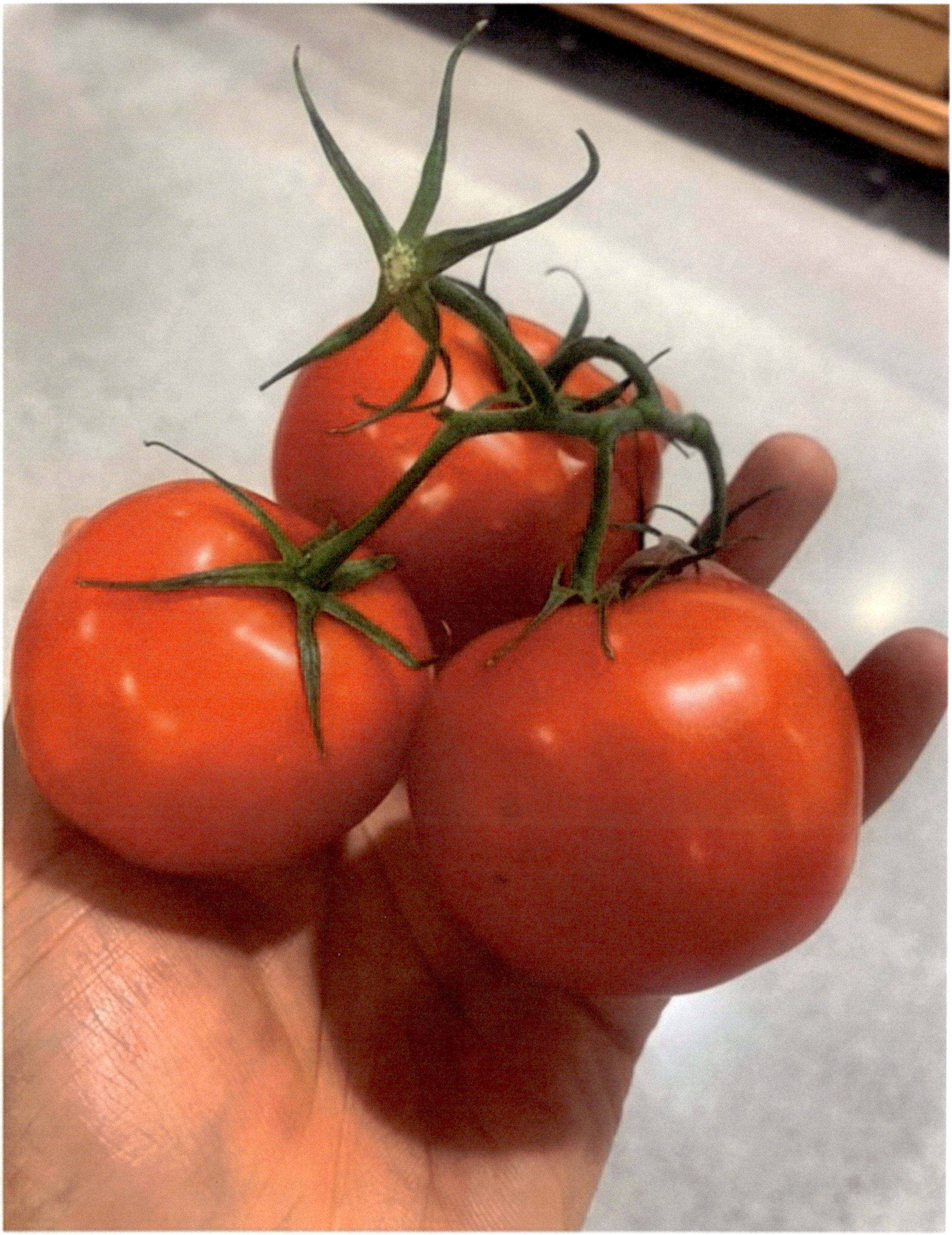

VITAMIN B

Bananas

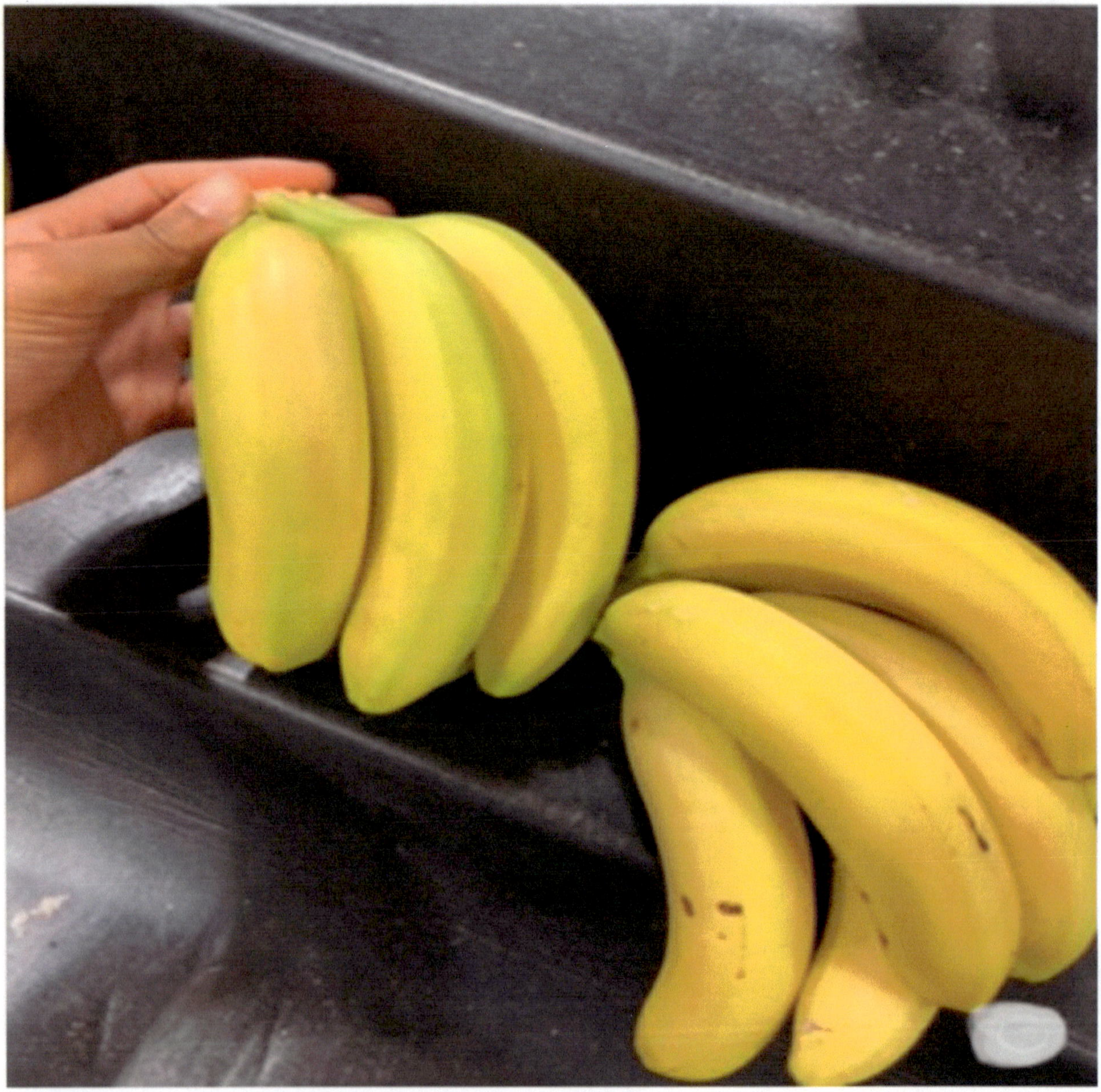

Bananas (peeled)

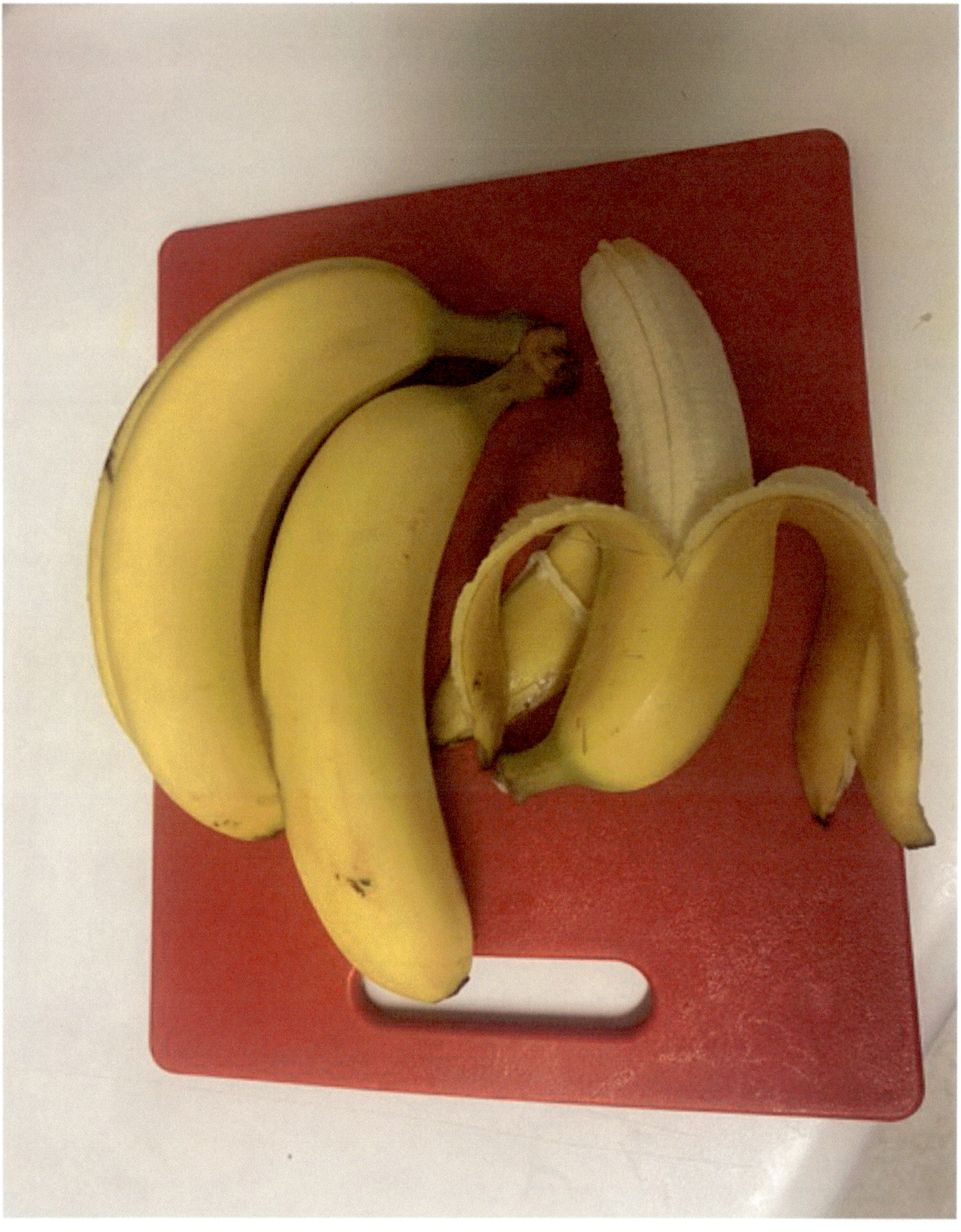

Pineapple

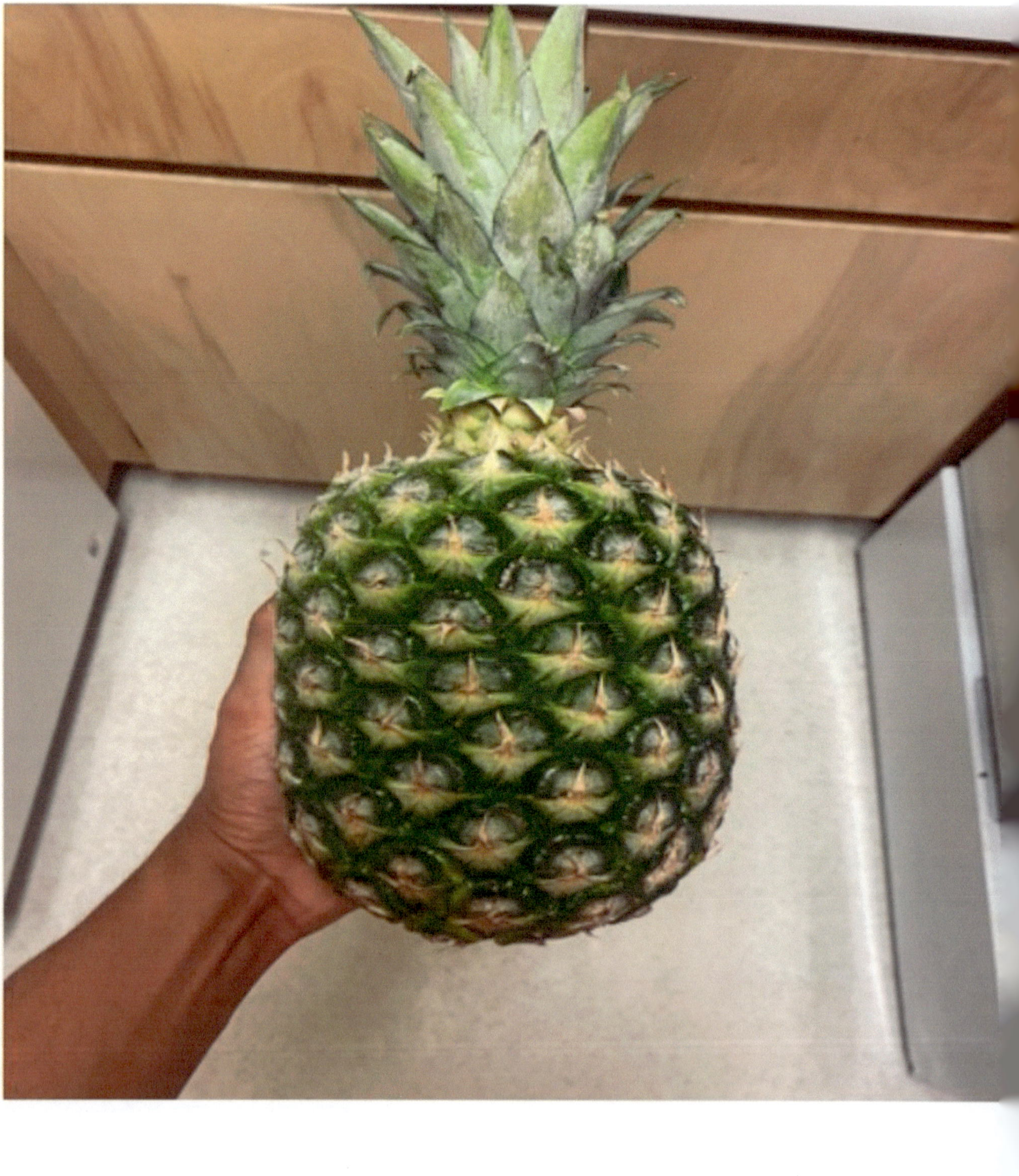

Pineapple (Sliced)

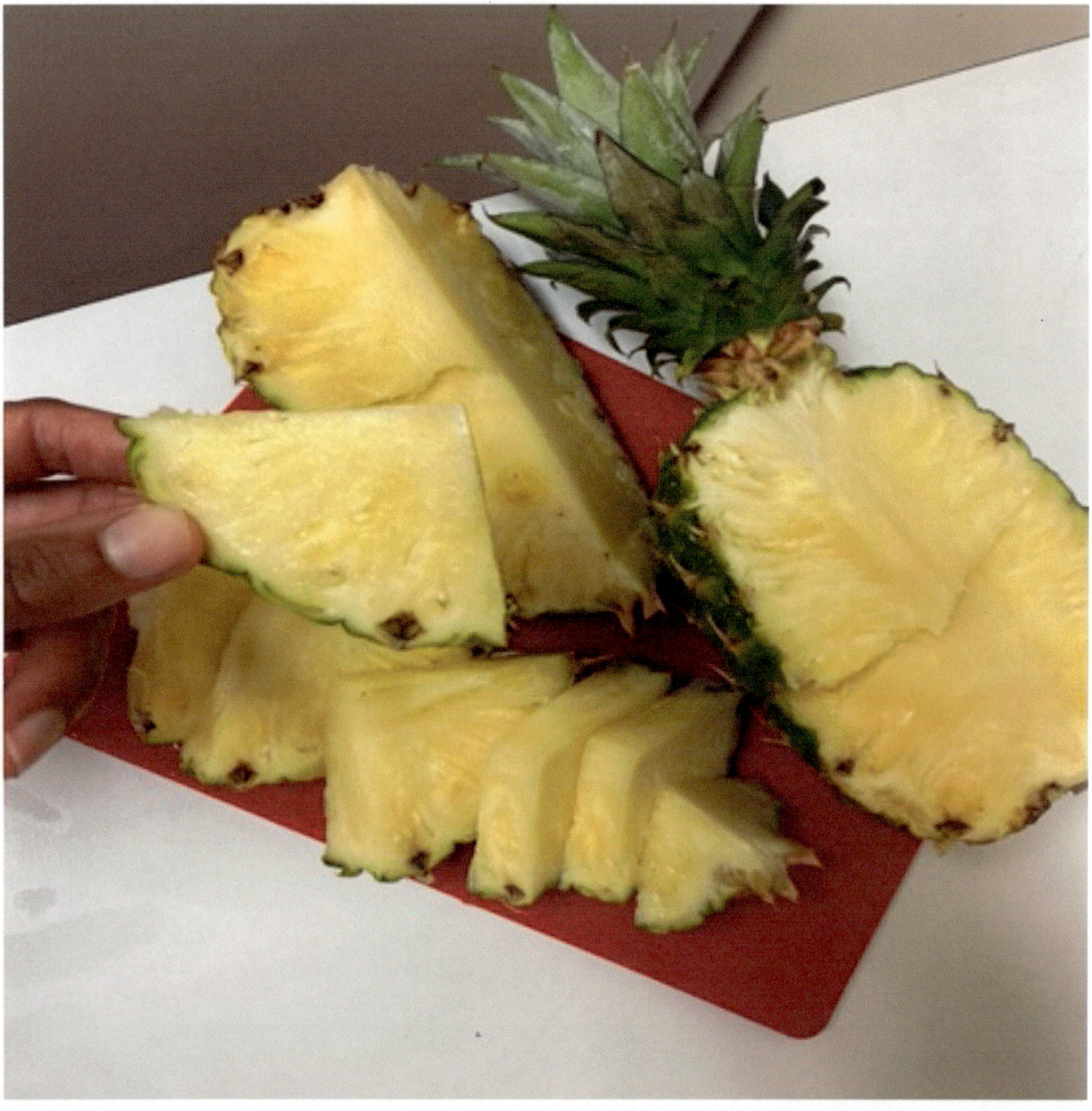

Green Beans

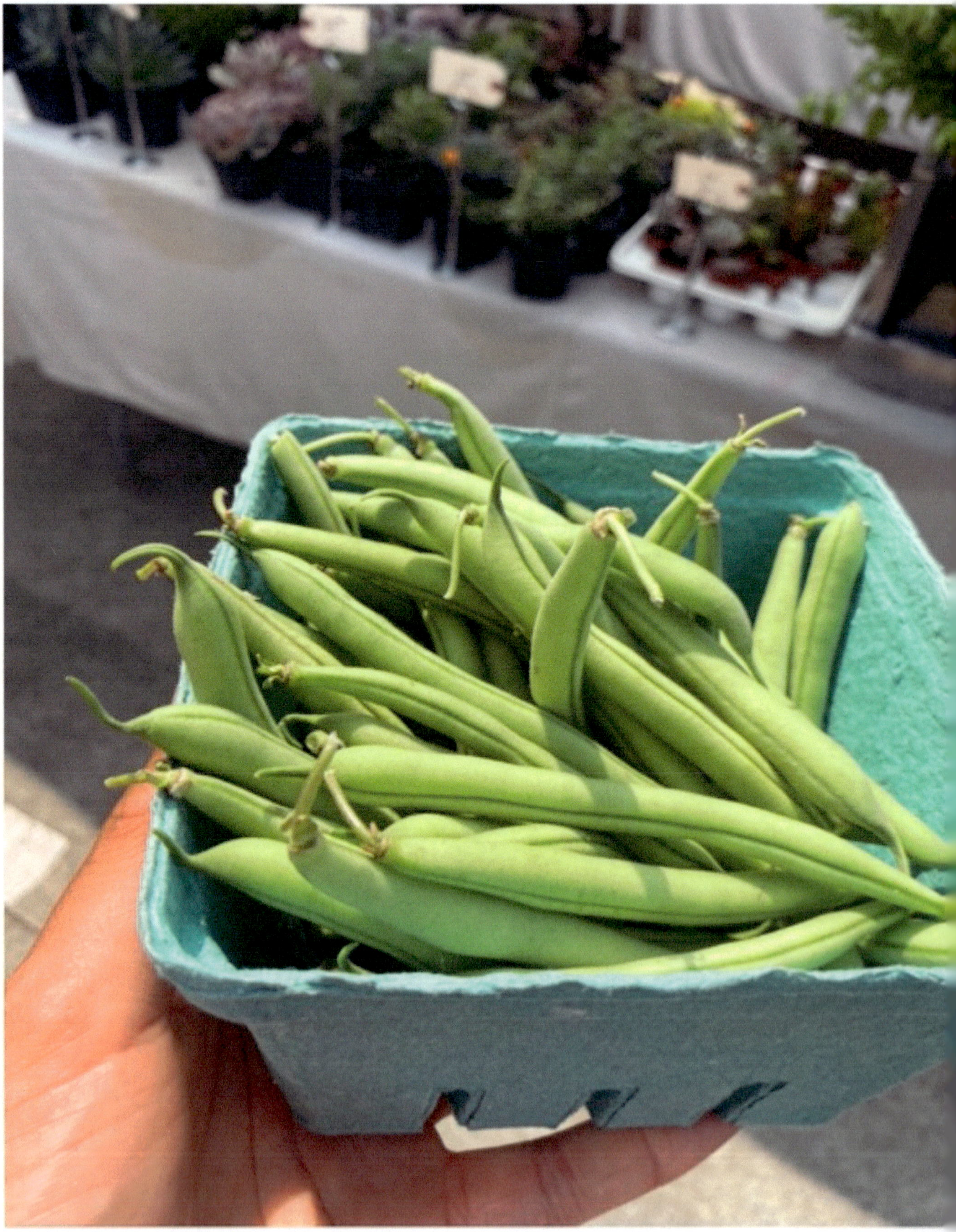

Black beans (top)

Red Beans (Bottom)

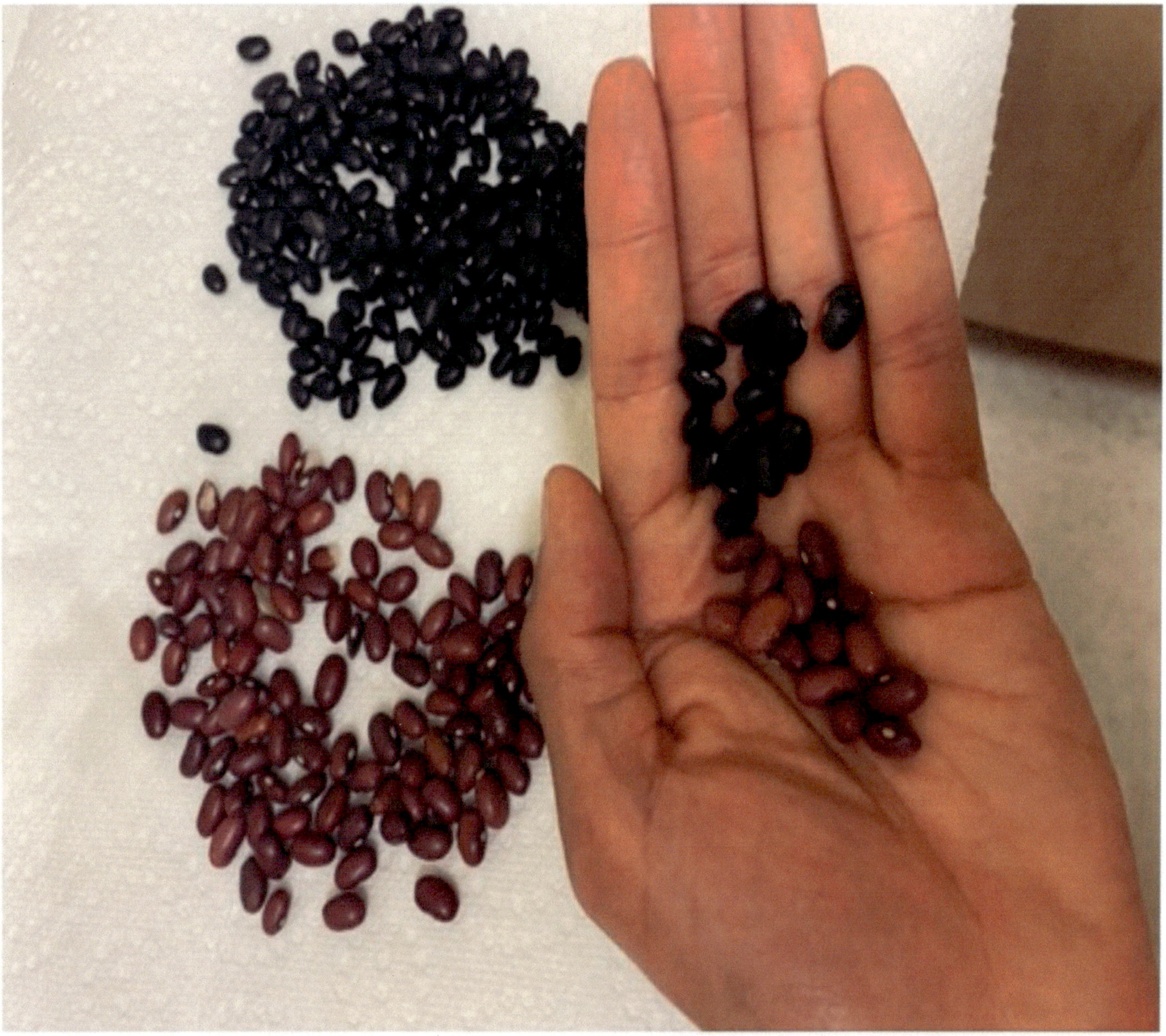

Popcorn

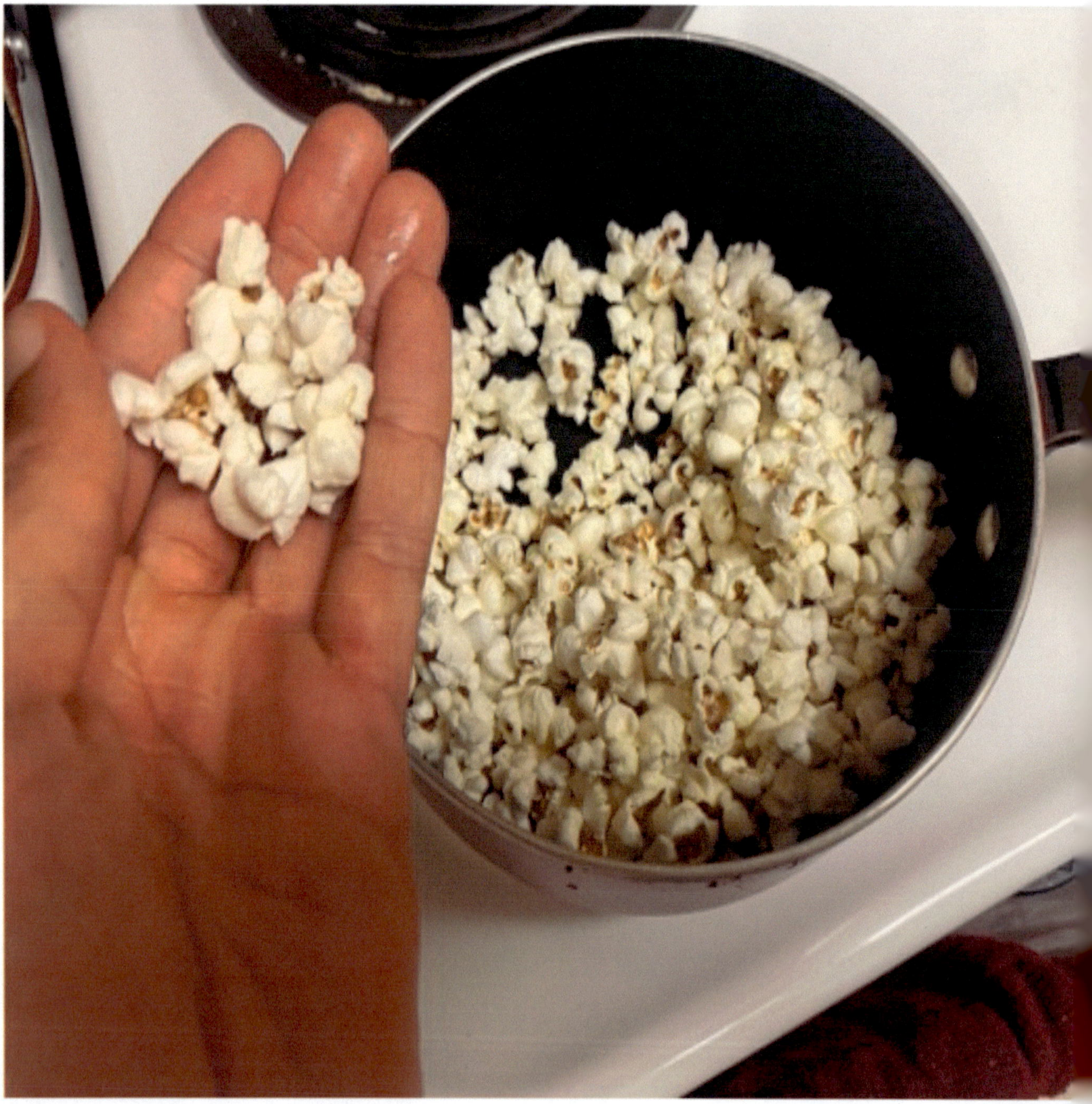

VITAMIN C

Red grapes (*with seeds*)

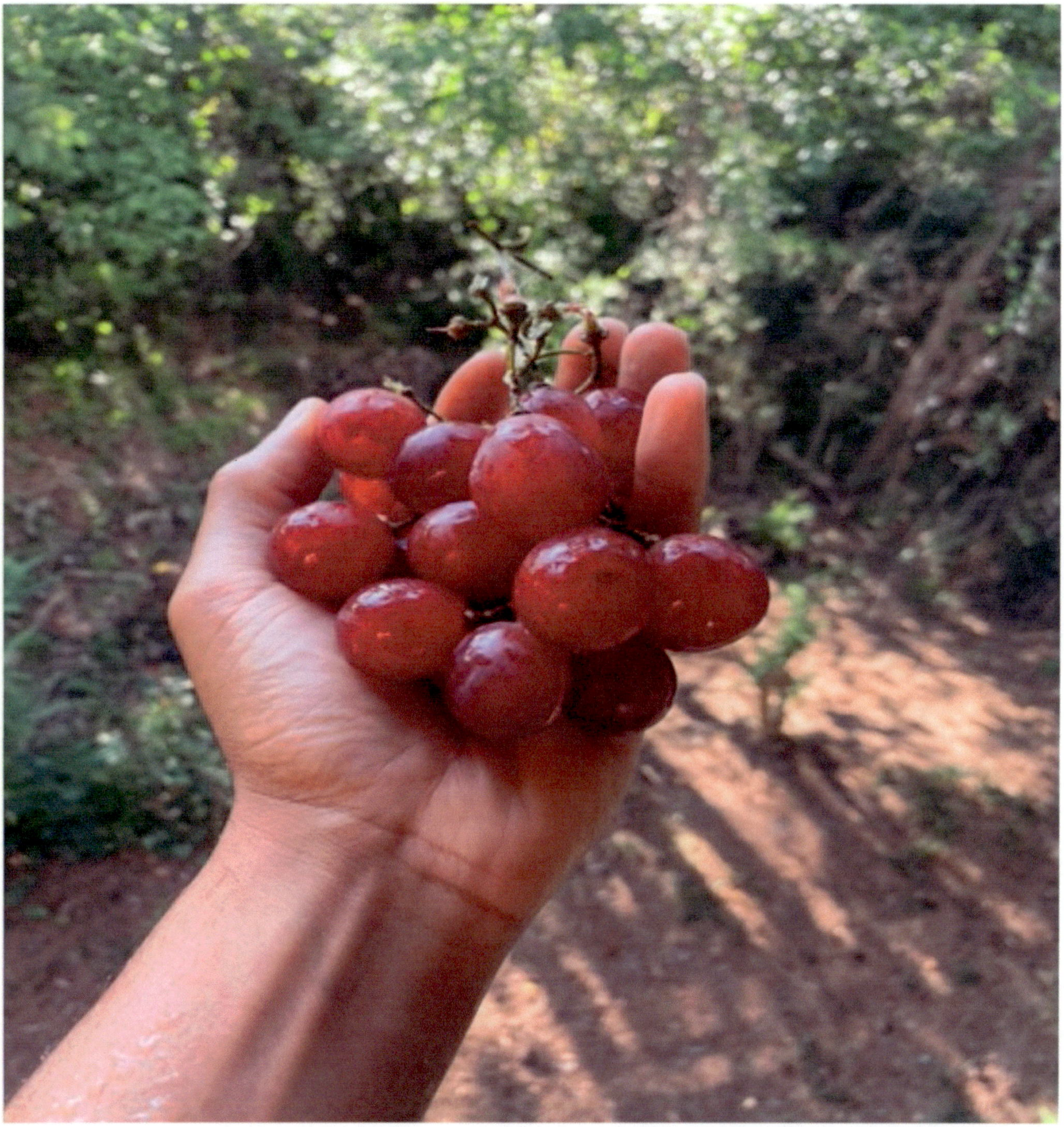

Strawberries

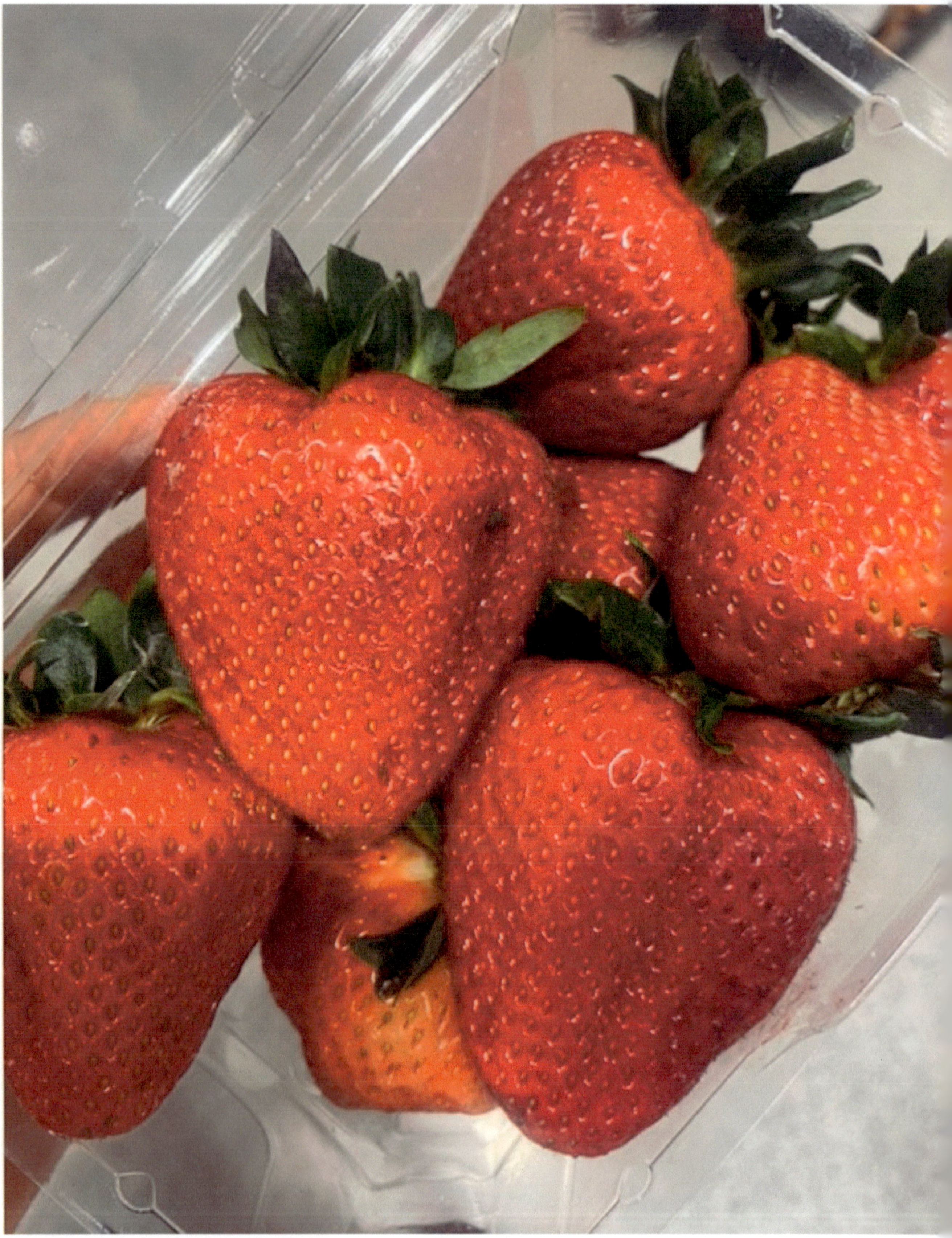

Blue Berries

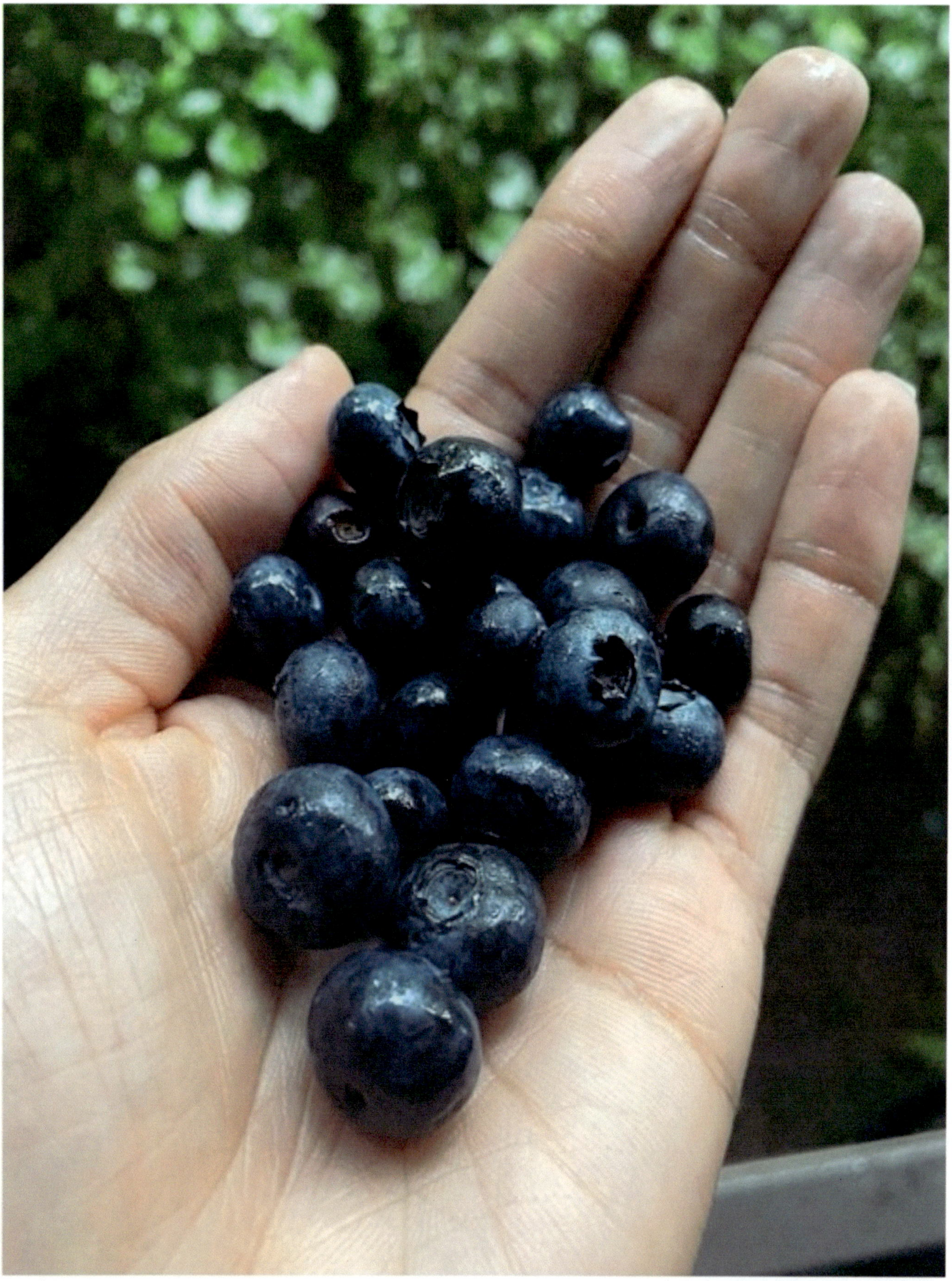

Oranges

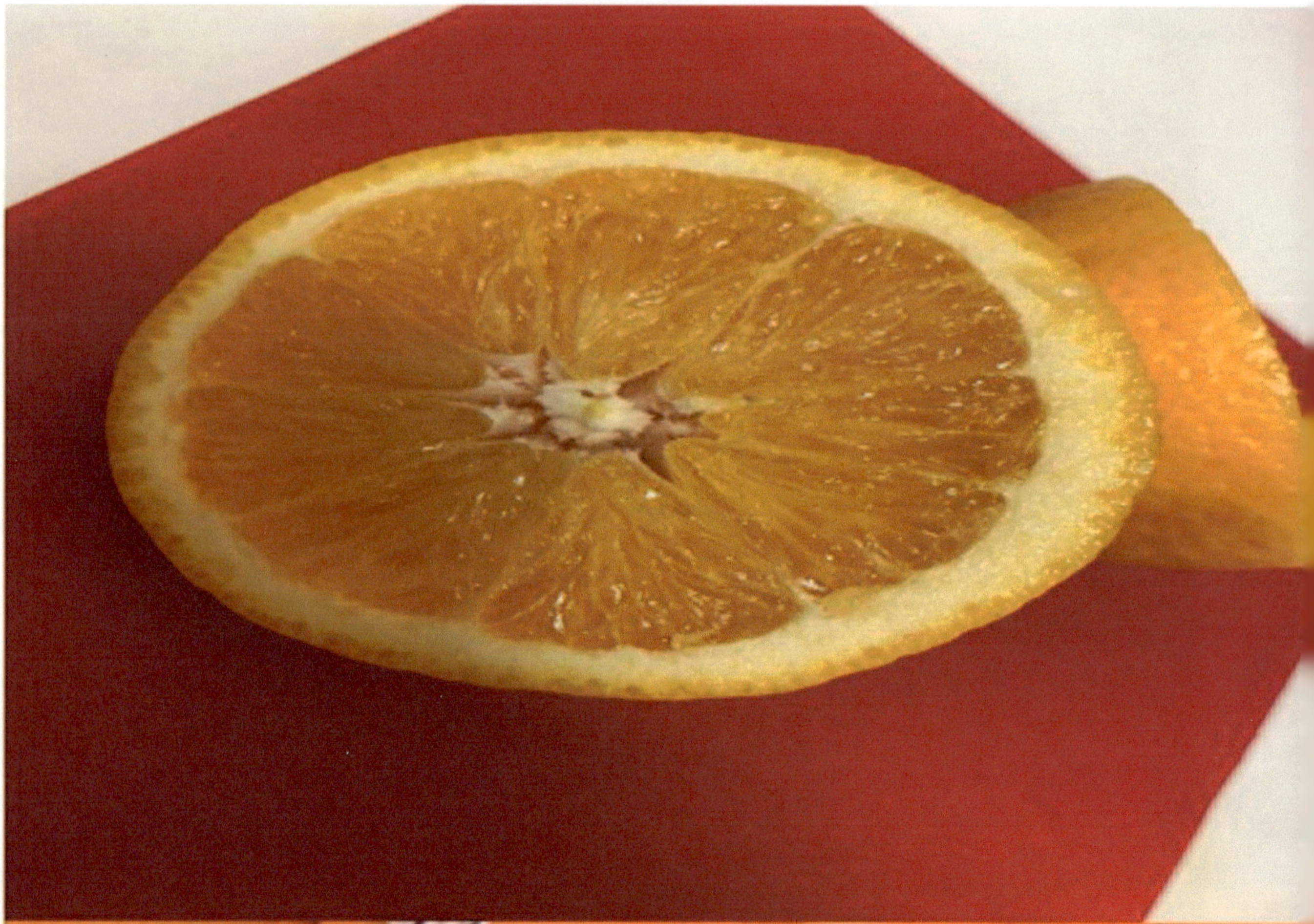

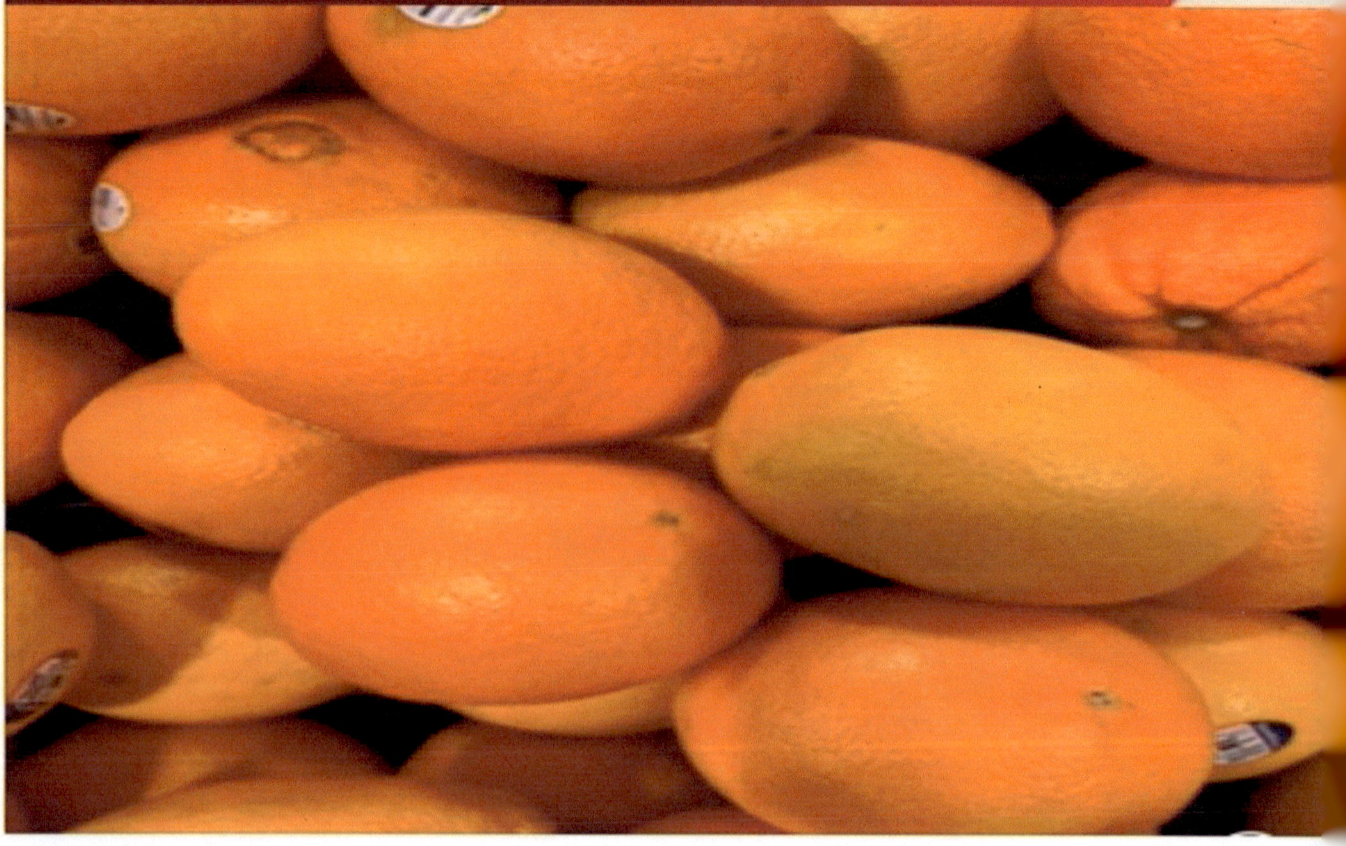

VITAMIN D

Mushrooms

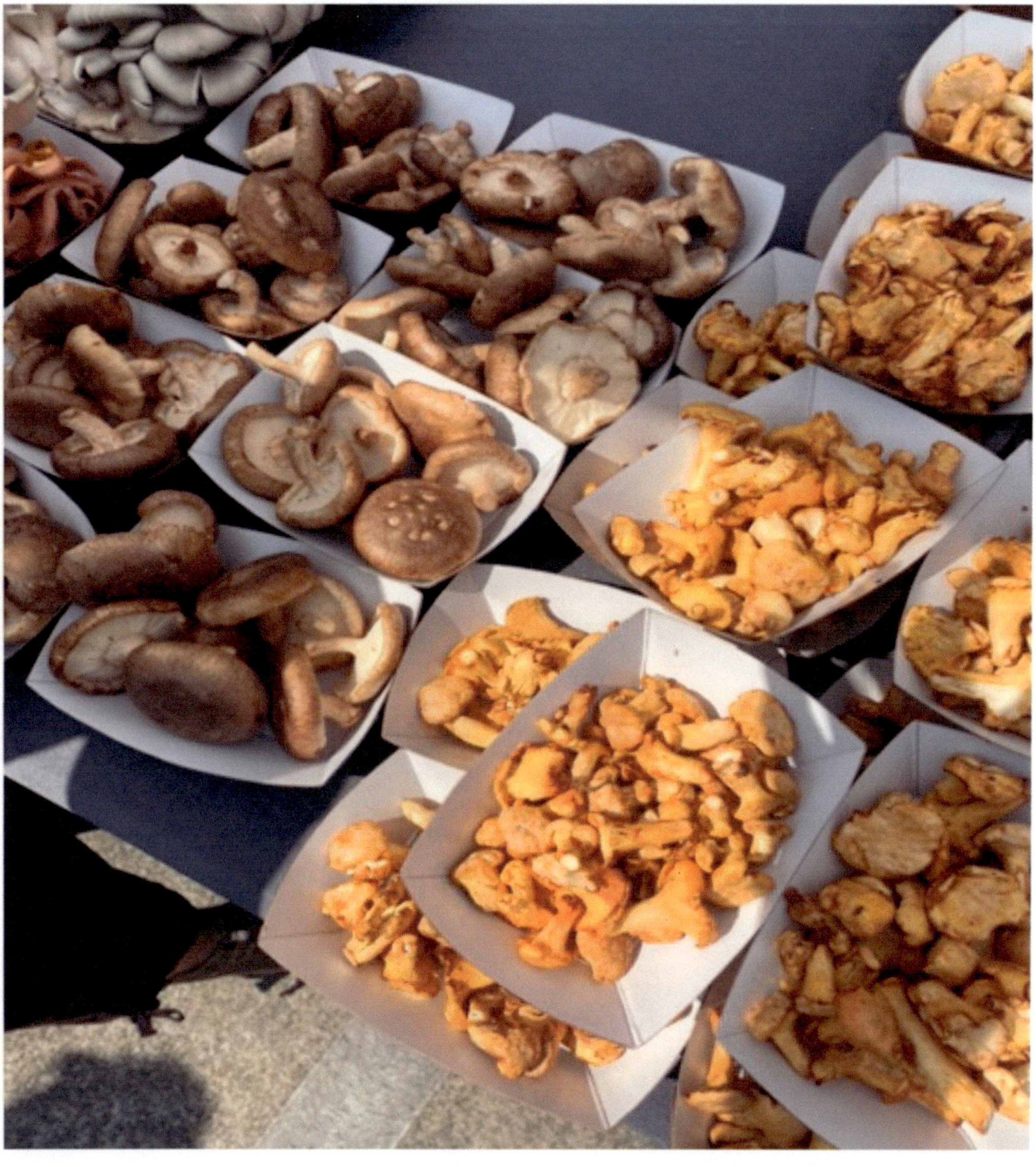

Sunshine on the pier

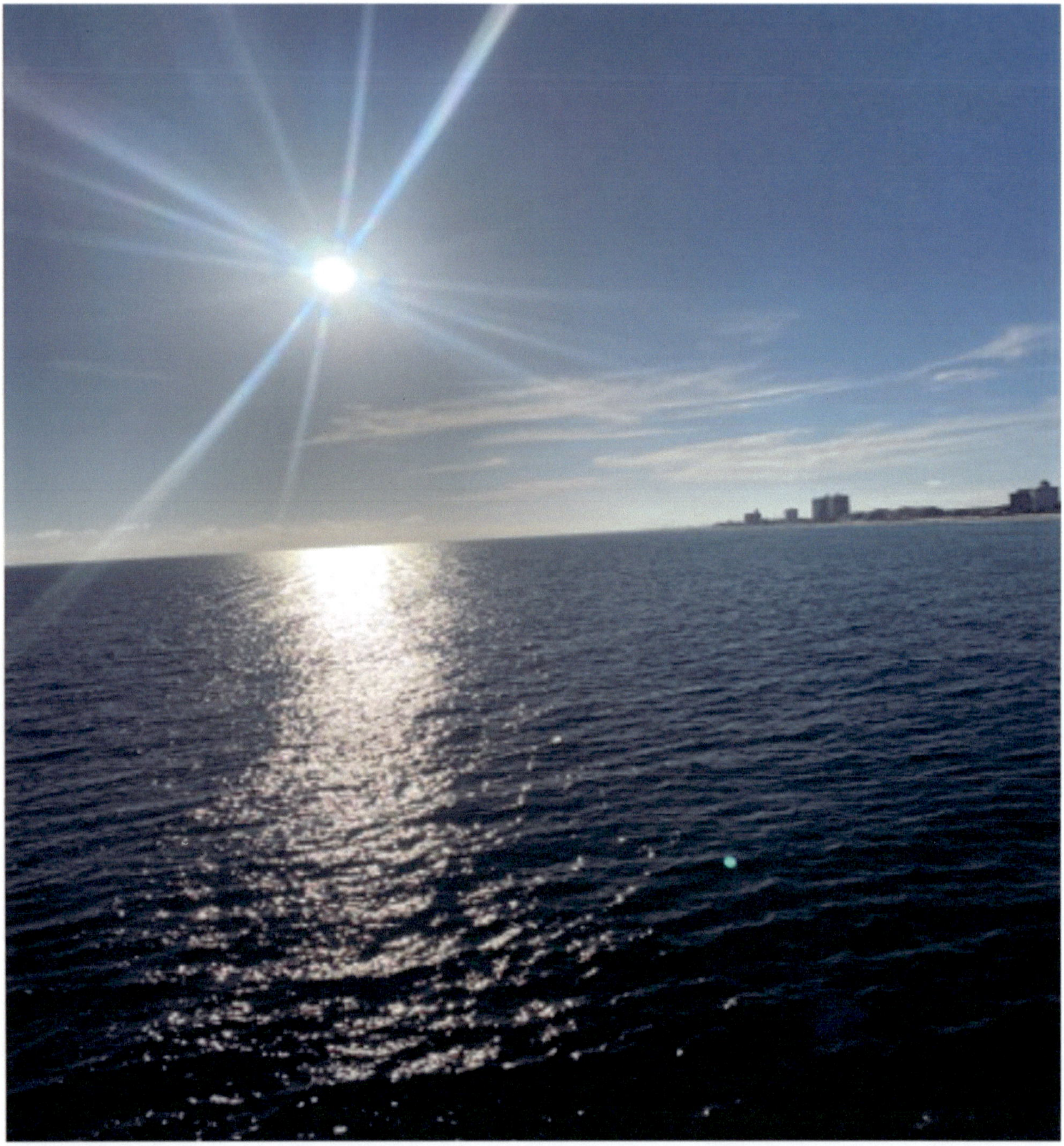

Sunshine at the park under the trees

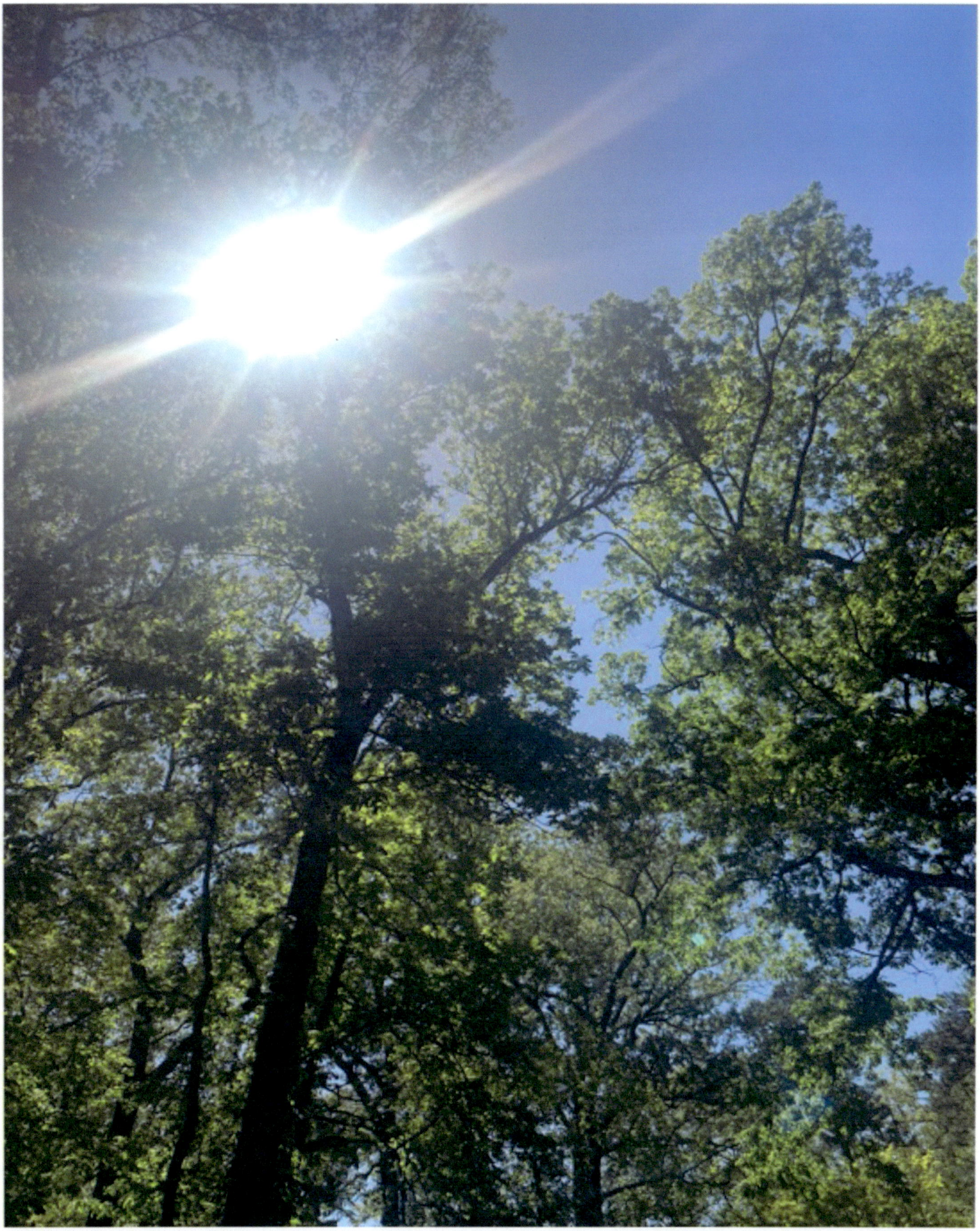

VITAMIN E

Sunflower Seeds

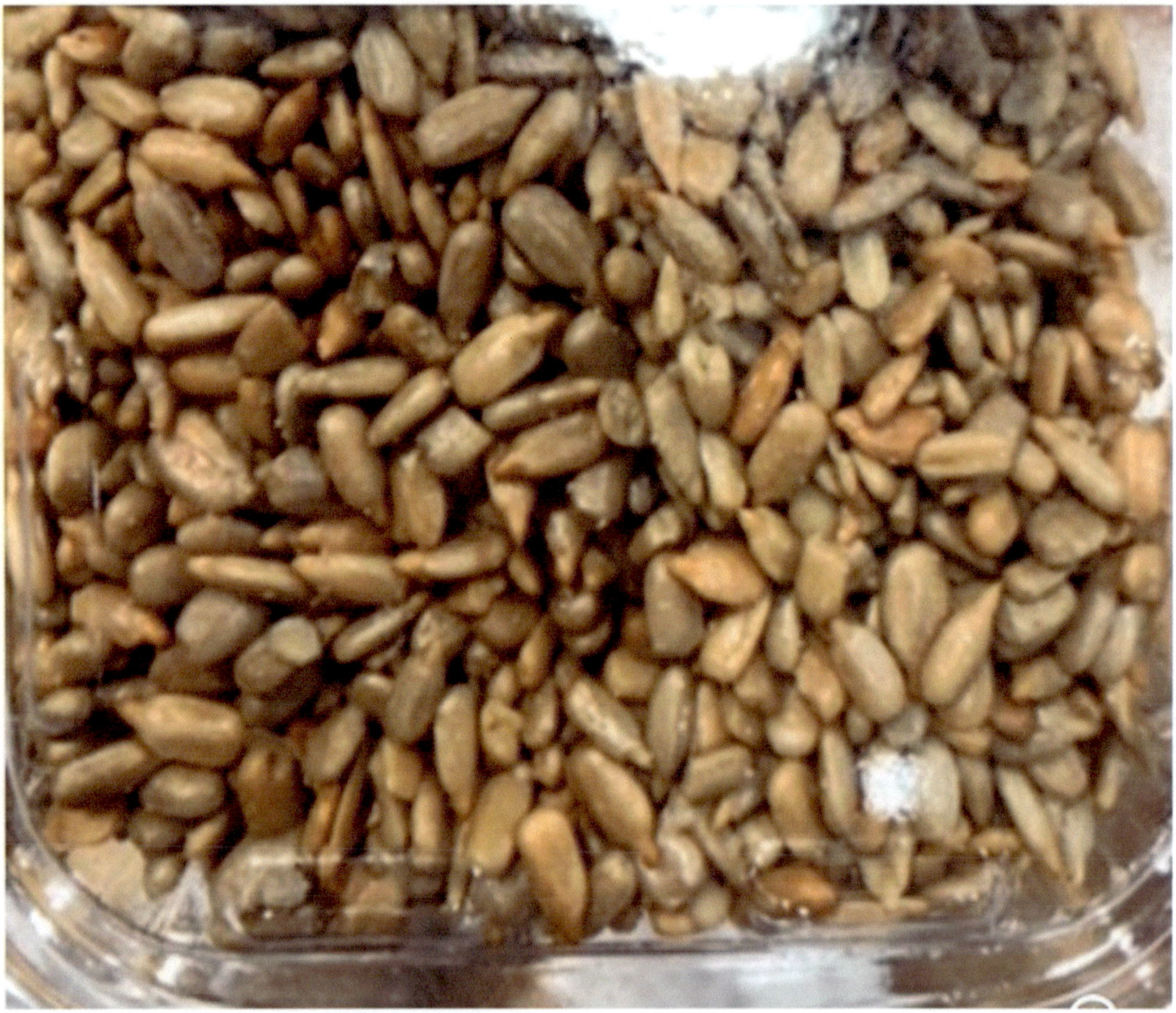

Almonds

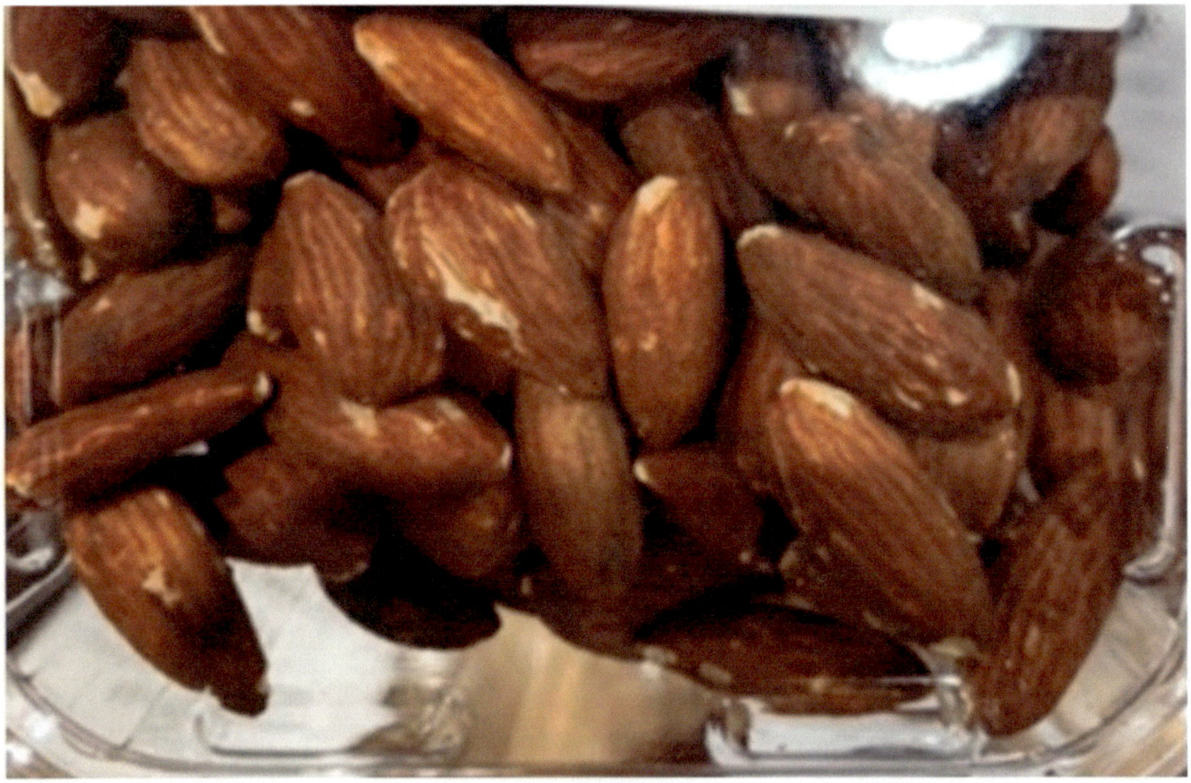

Sunflower Butter (also can be a substitute for peanut butter)

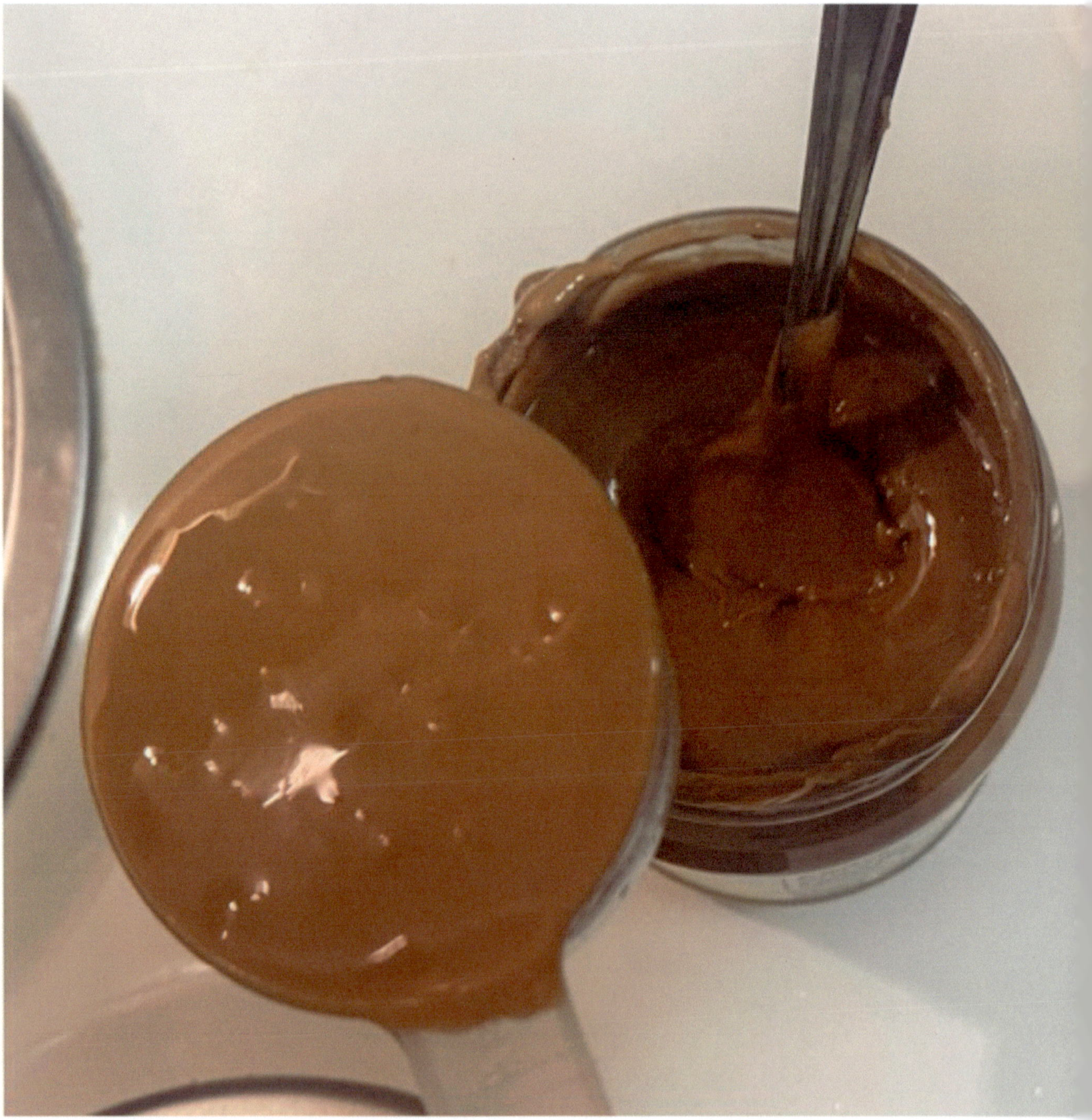

VITAMIN K

Parsley

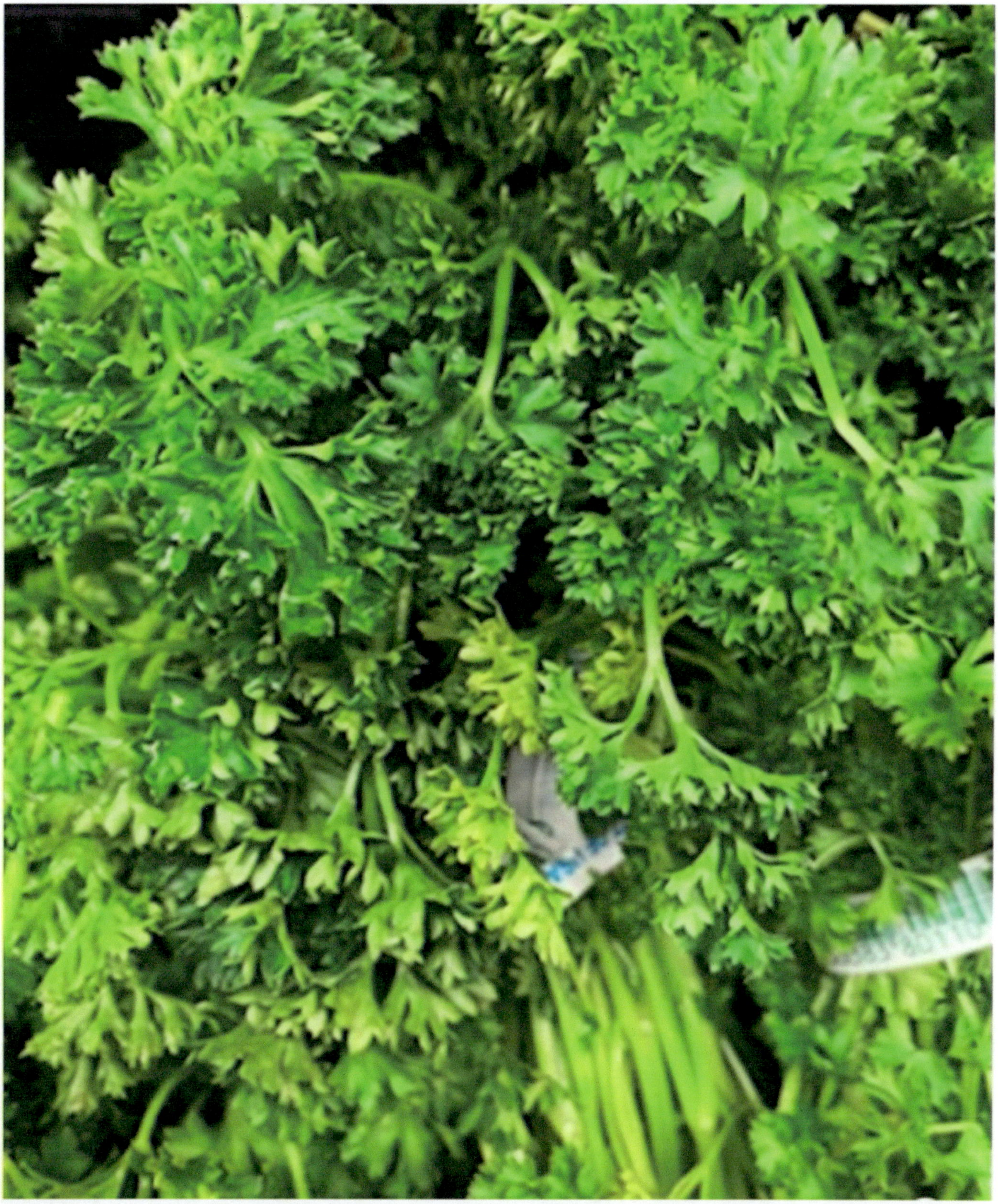

Kale

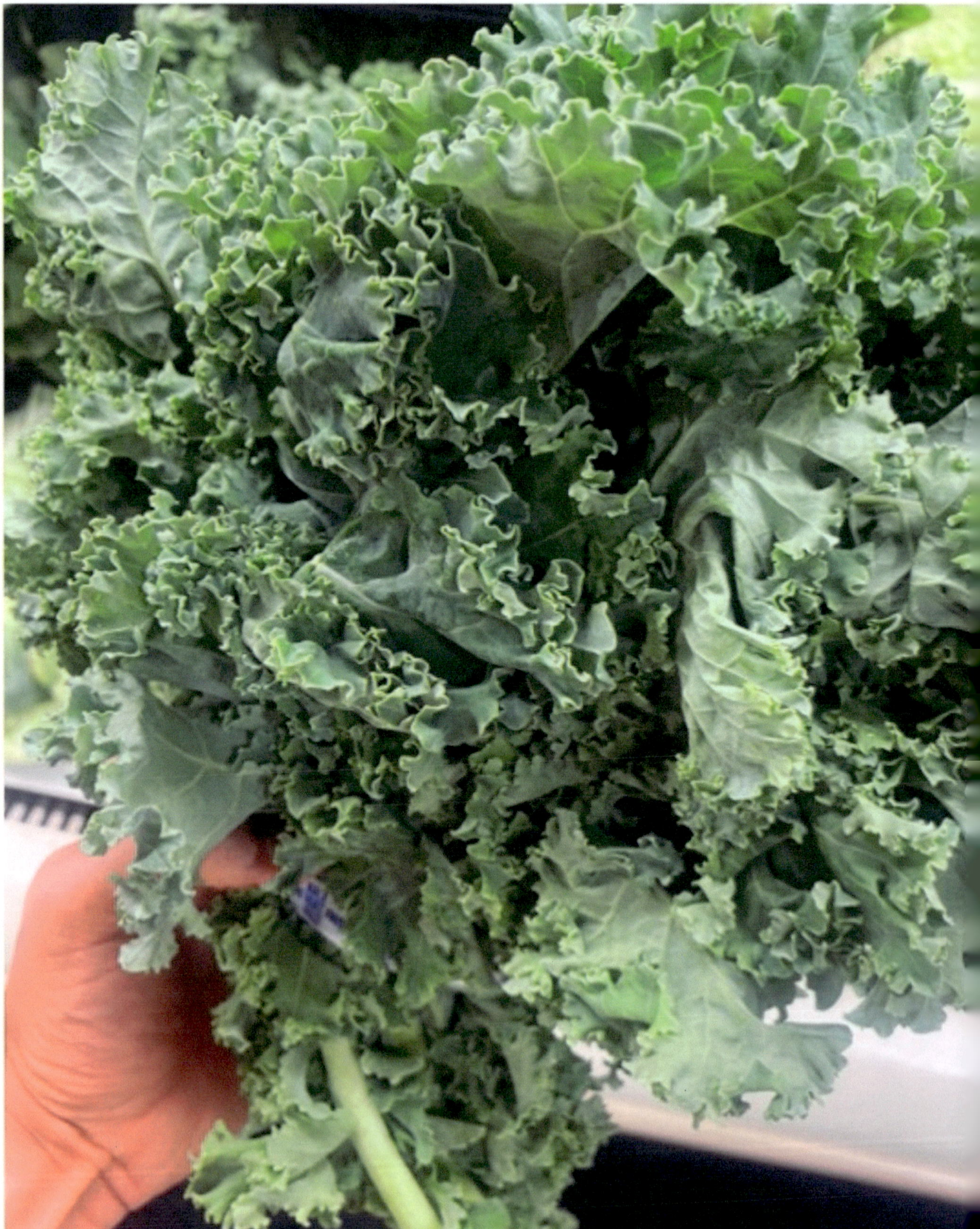

Collards

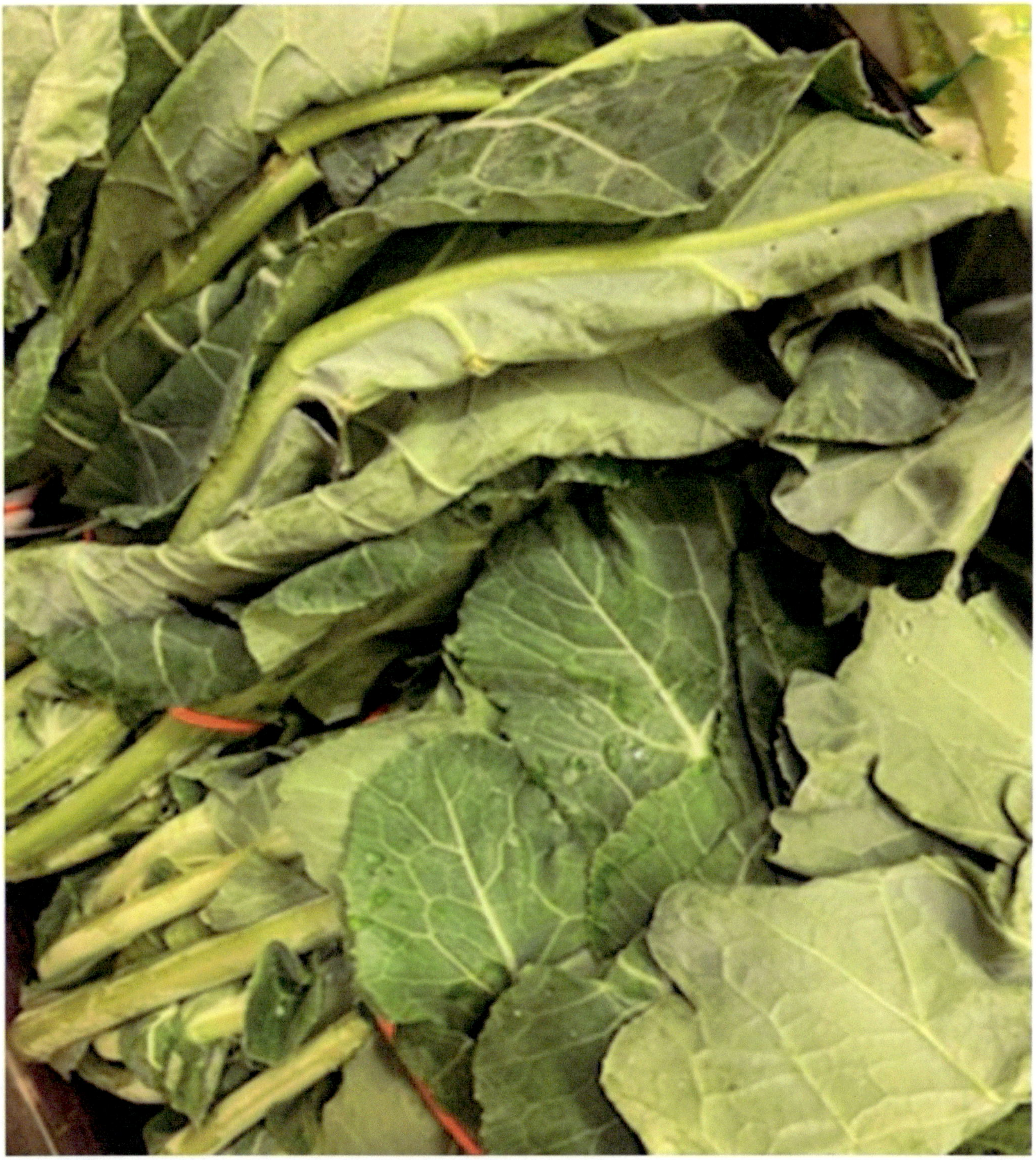

Bonus Material 2

Miscellaneous photos from the market and farmers' market

Peaches (left) Nectarines (right)

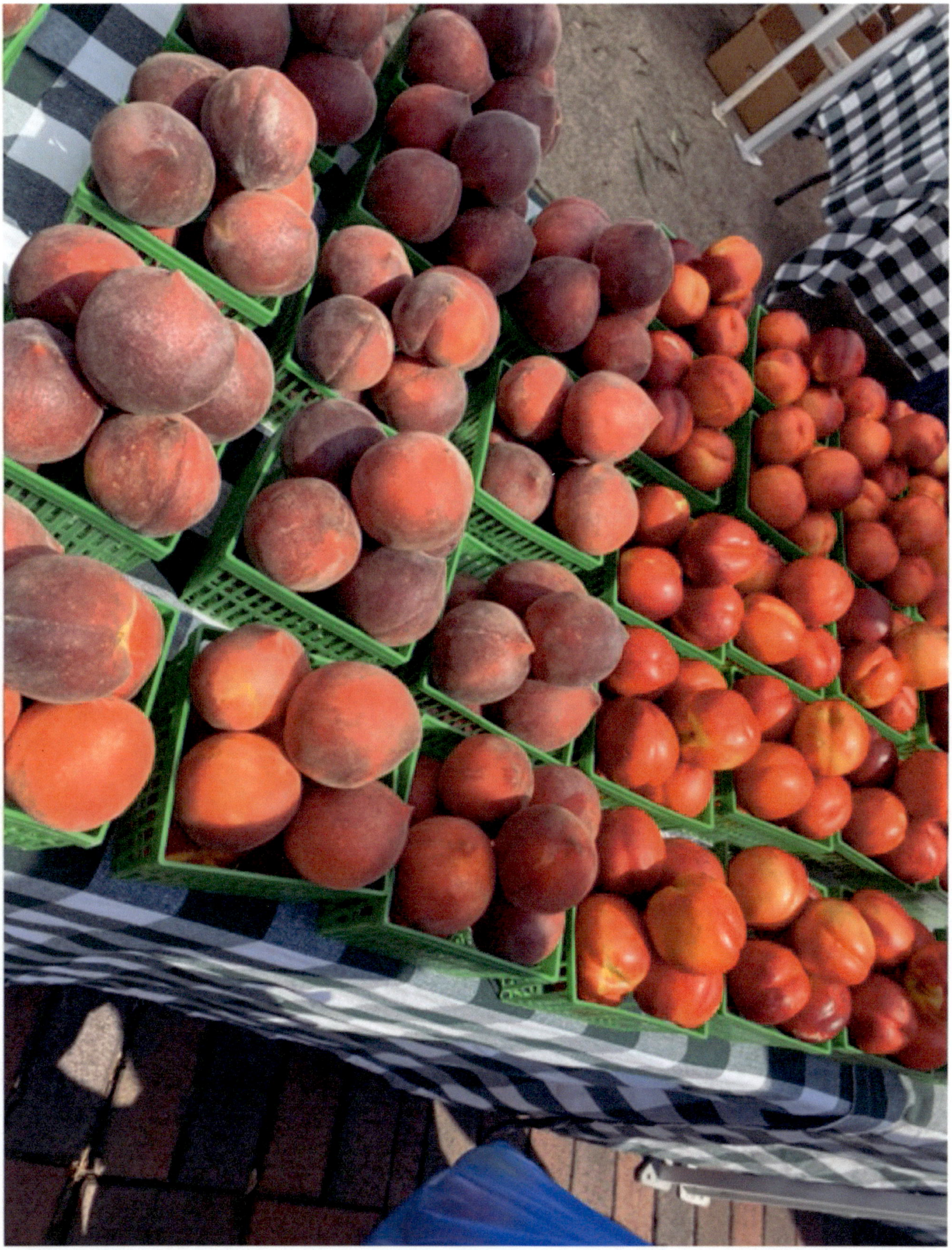

Blackberries

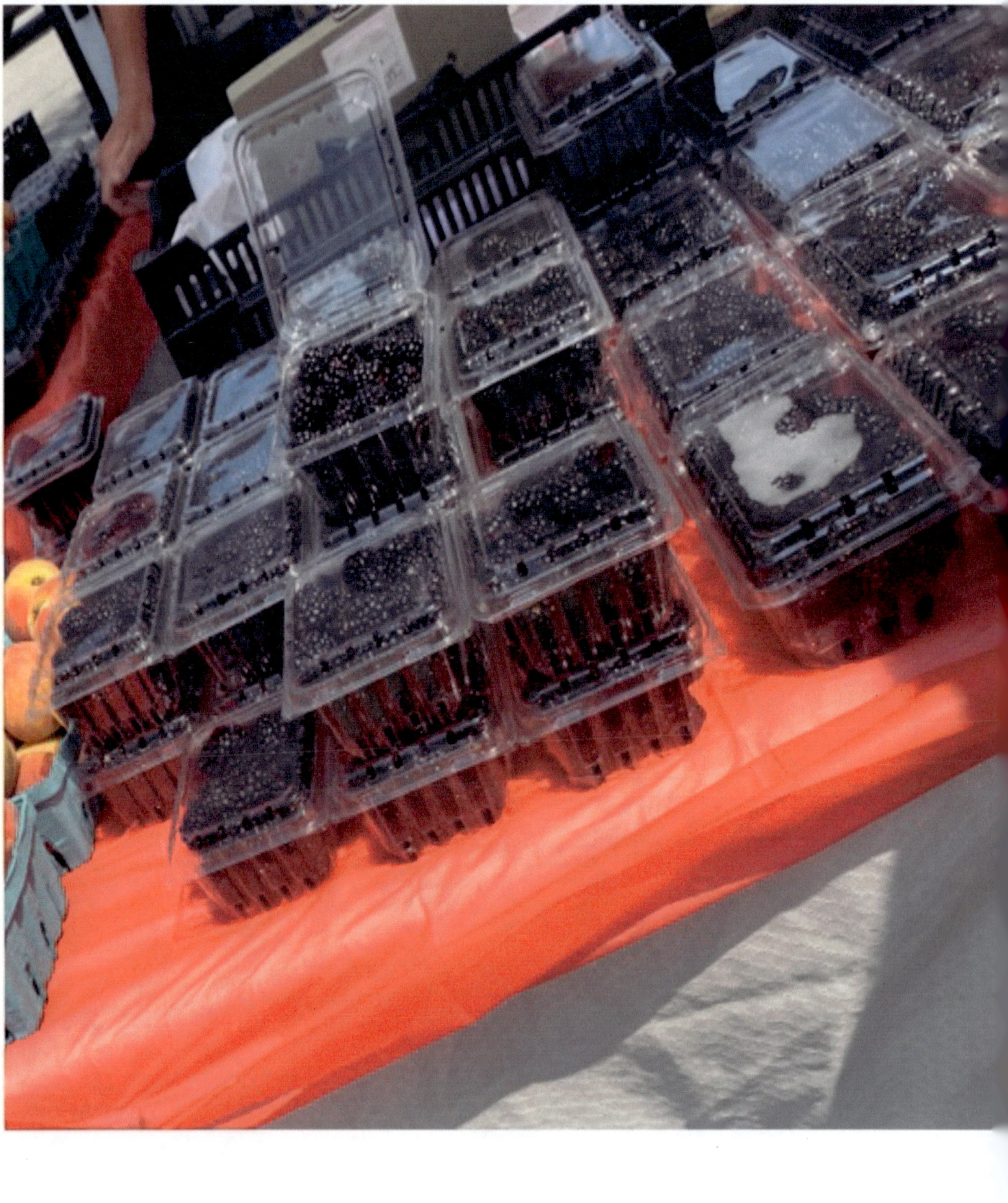

Carrots

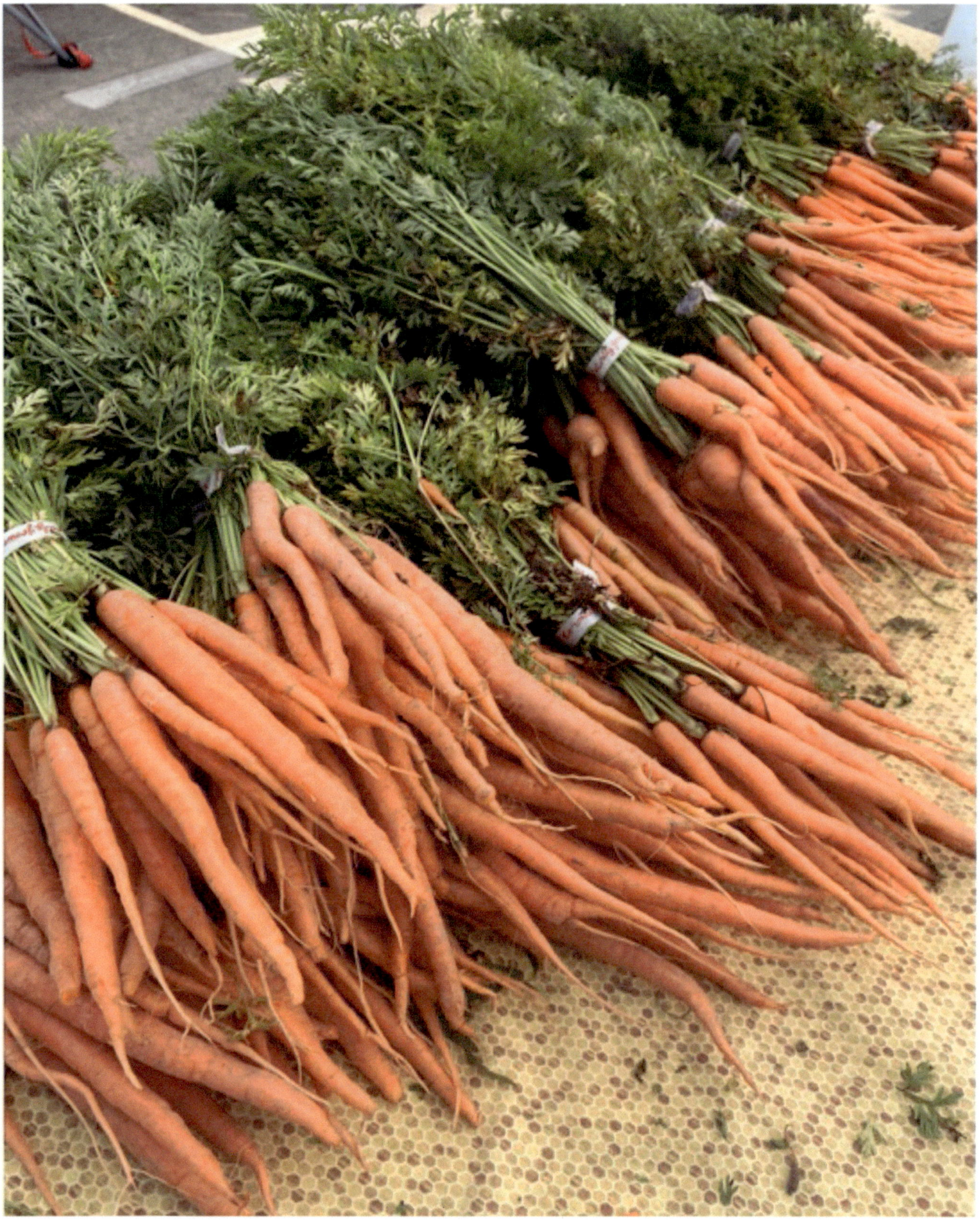

Squash and Zucchini

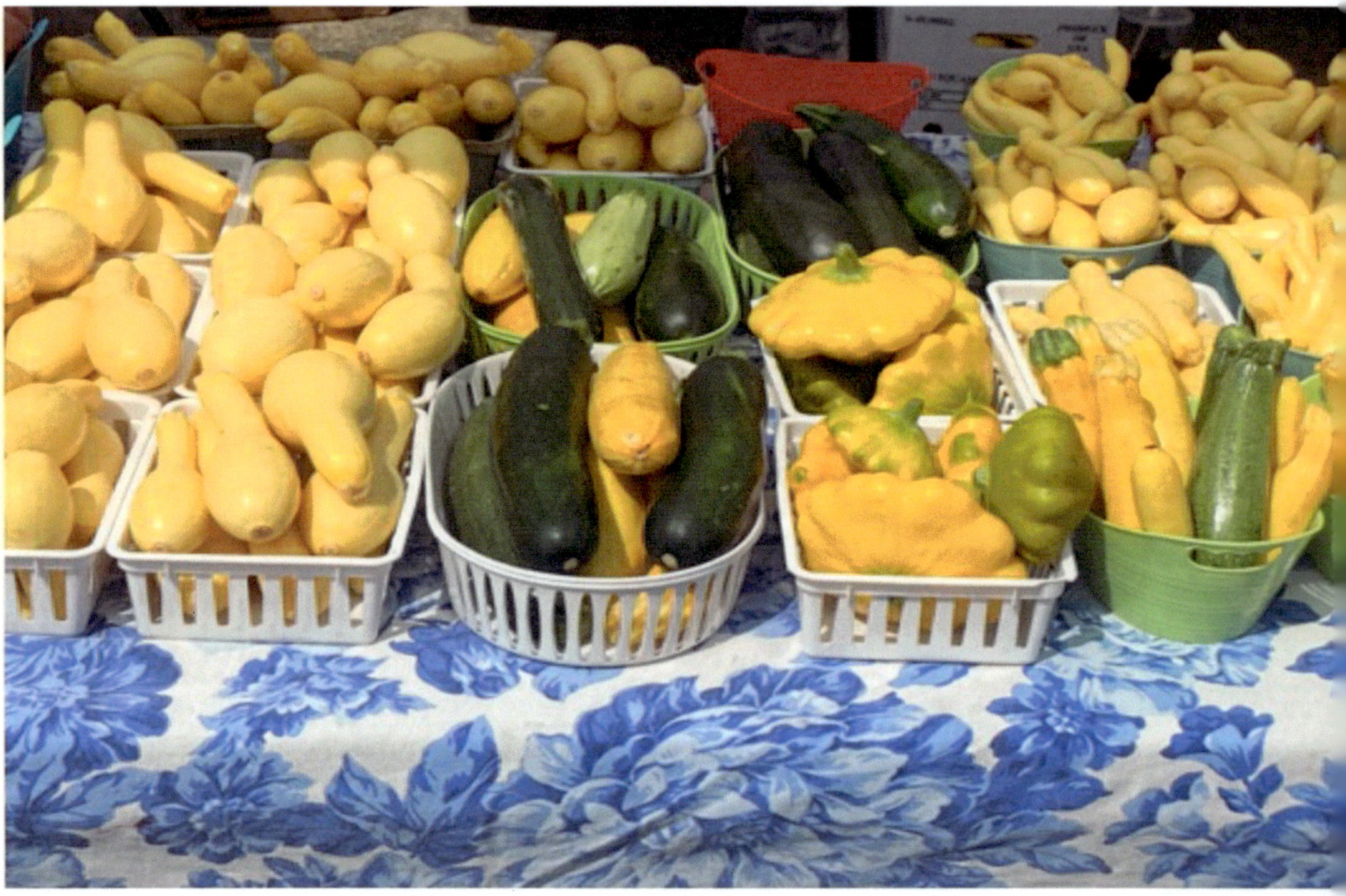

Blackberries, Strawberries, greengage plums, and red plums

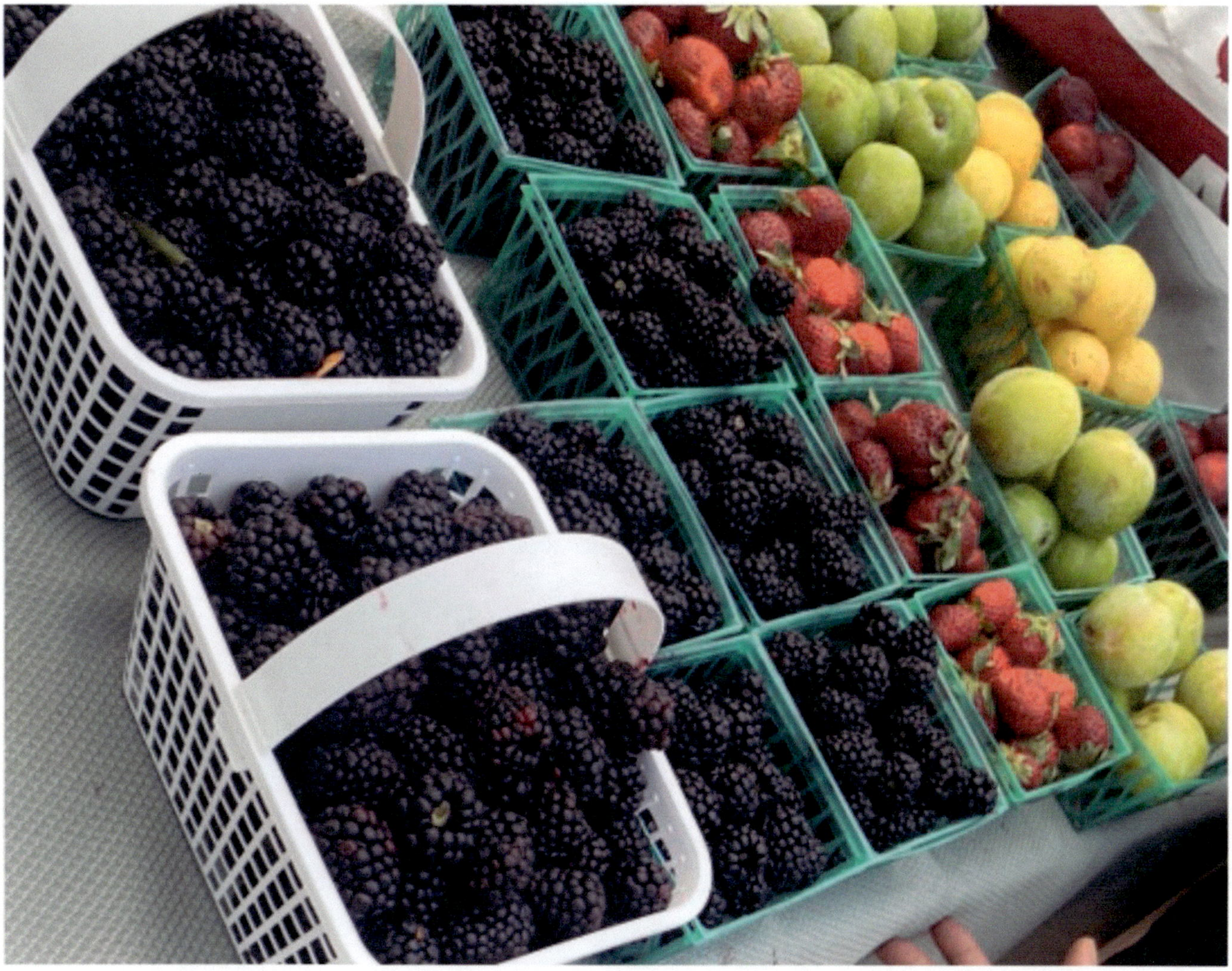

Sliced white onion, yellow bell pepper, Tomato, and green bell pepper

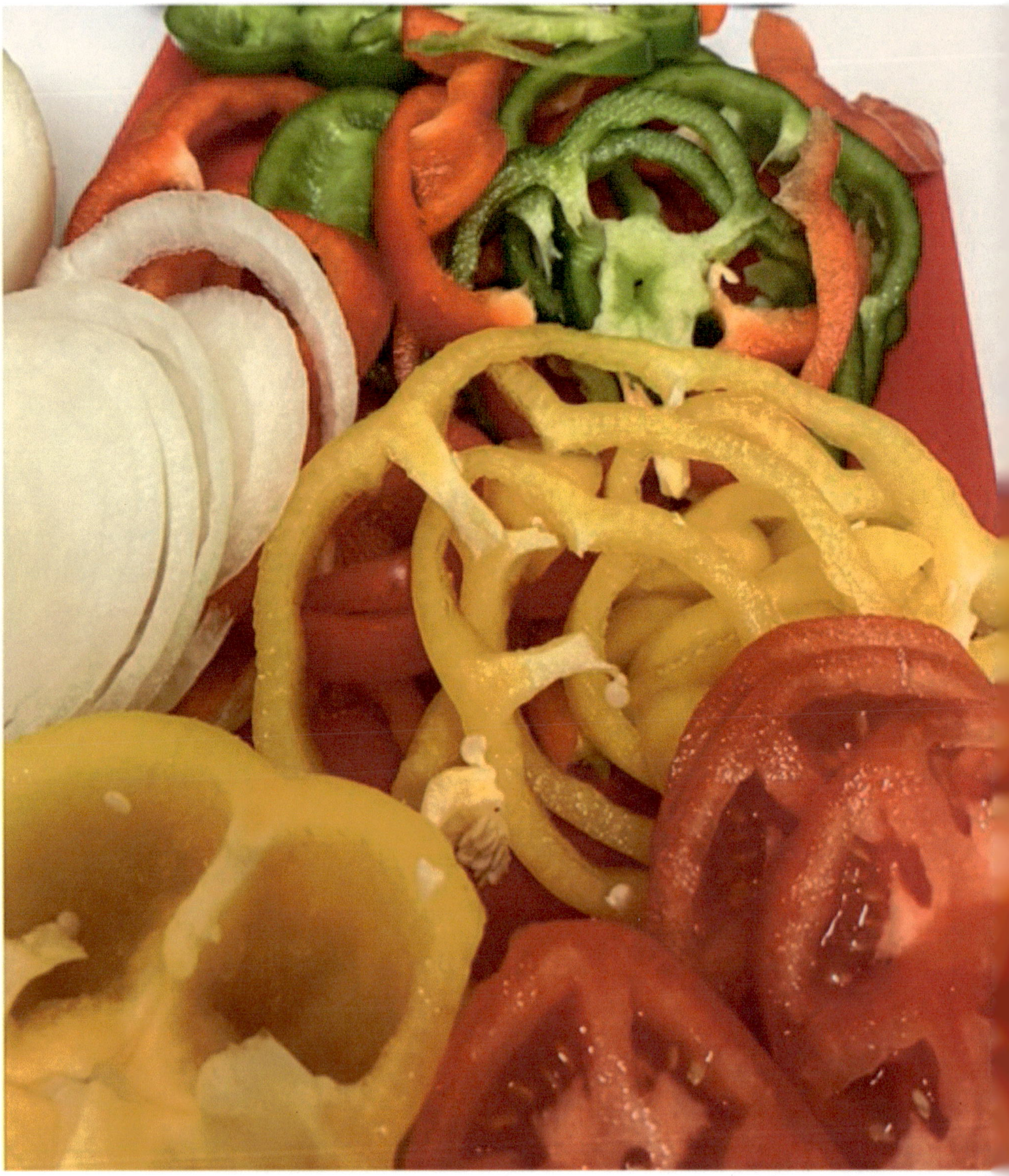

Jalapeño peppers *spicy*

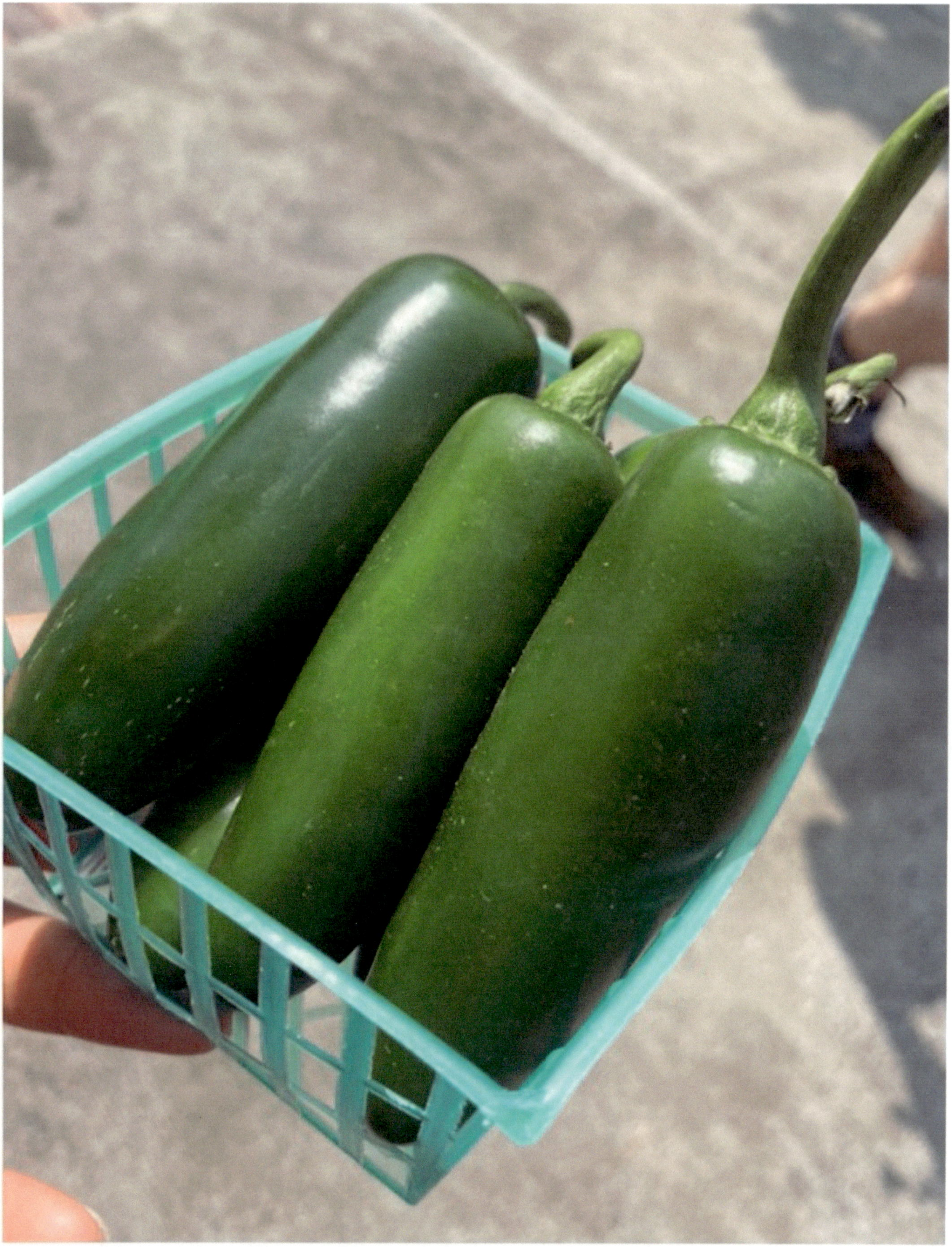

Carambola (also called Star fruit) (left), White dragon fruit (Center), yellow dragon fruit (right

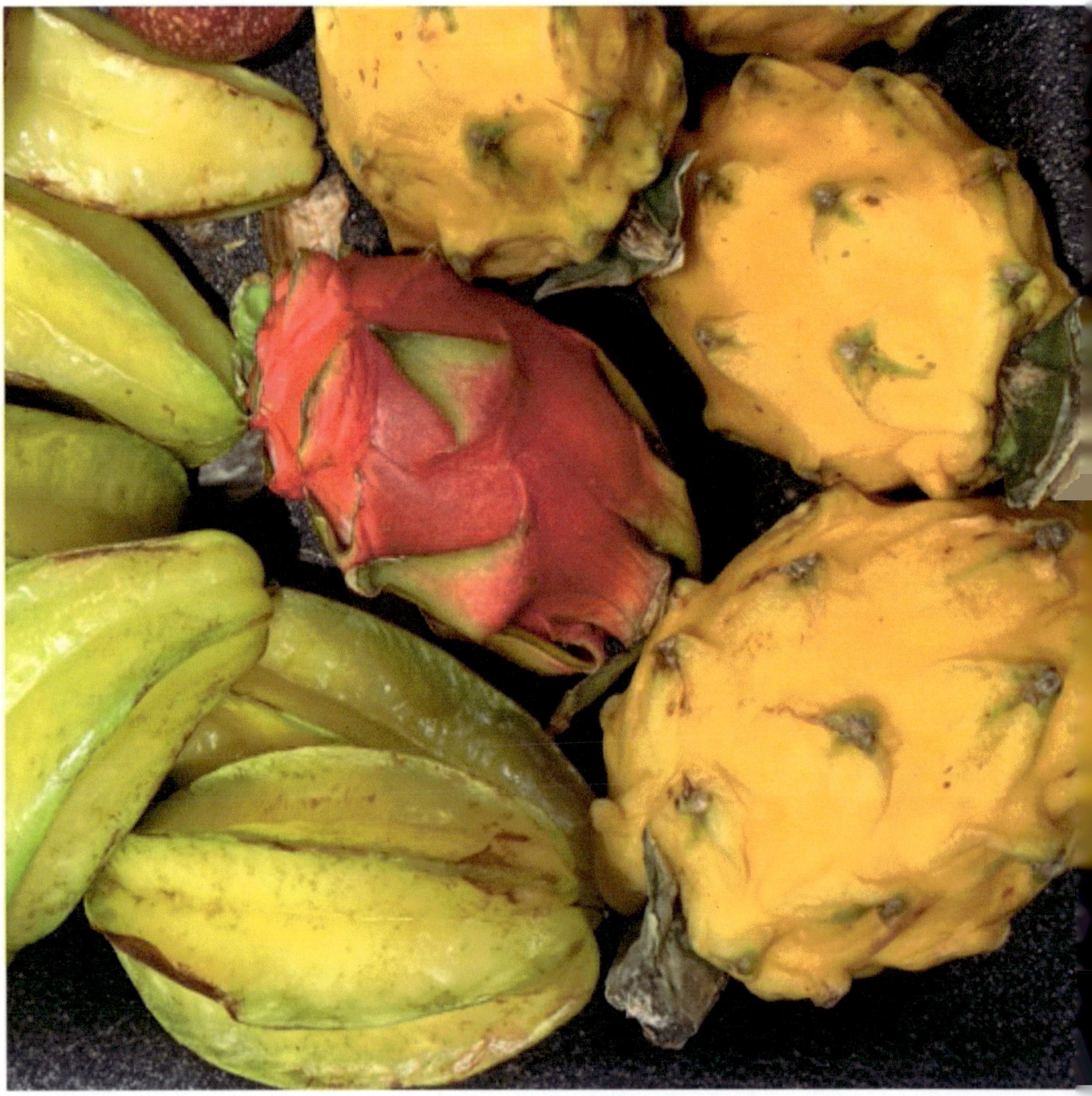

White dragon fruit (Sliced)

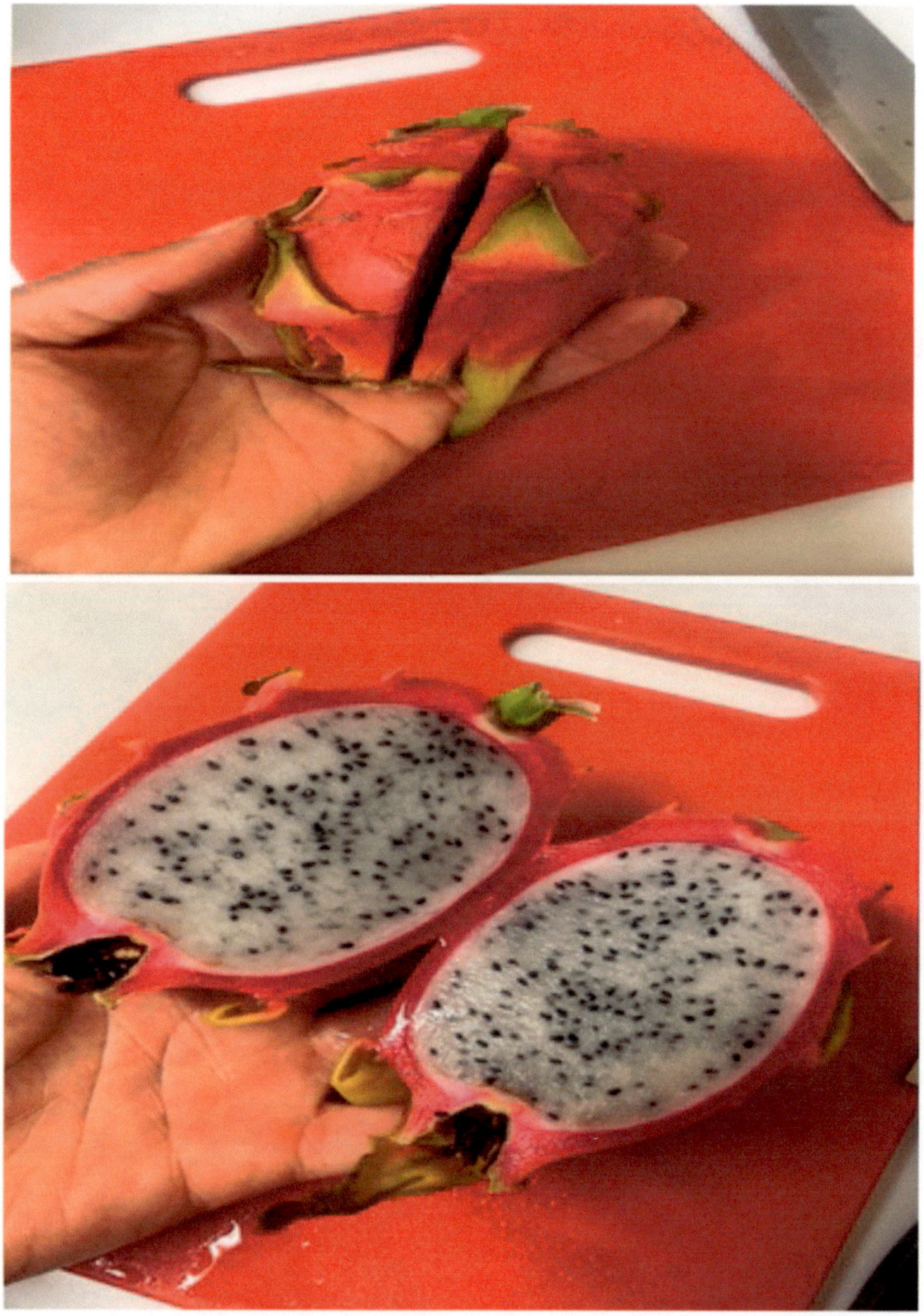

Starfruit (Carambola) (Sliced)

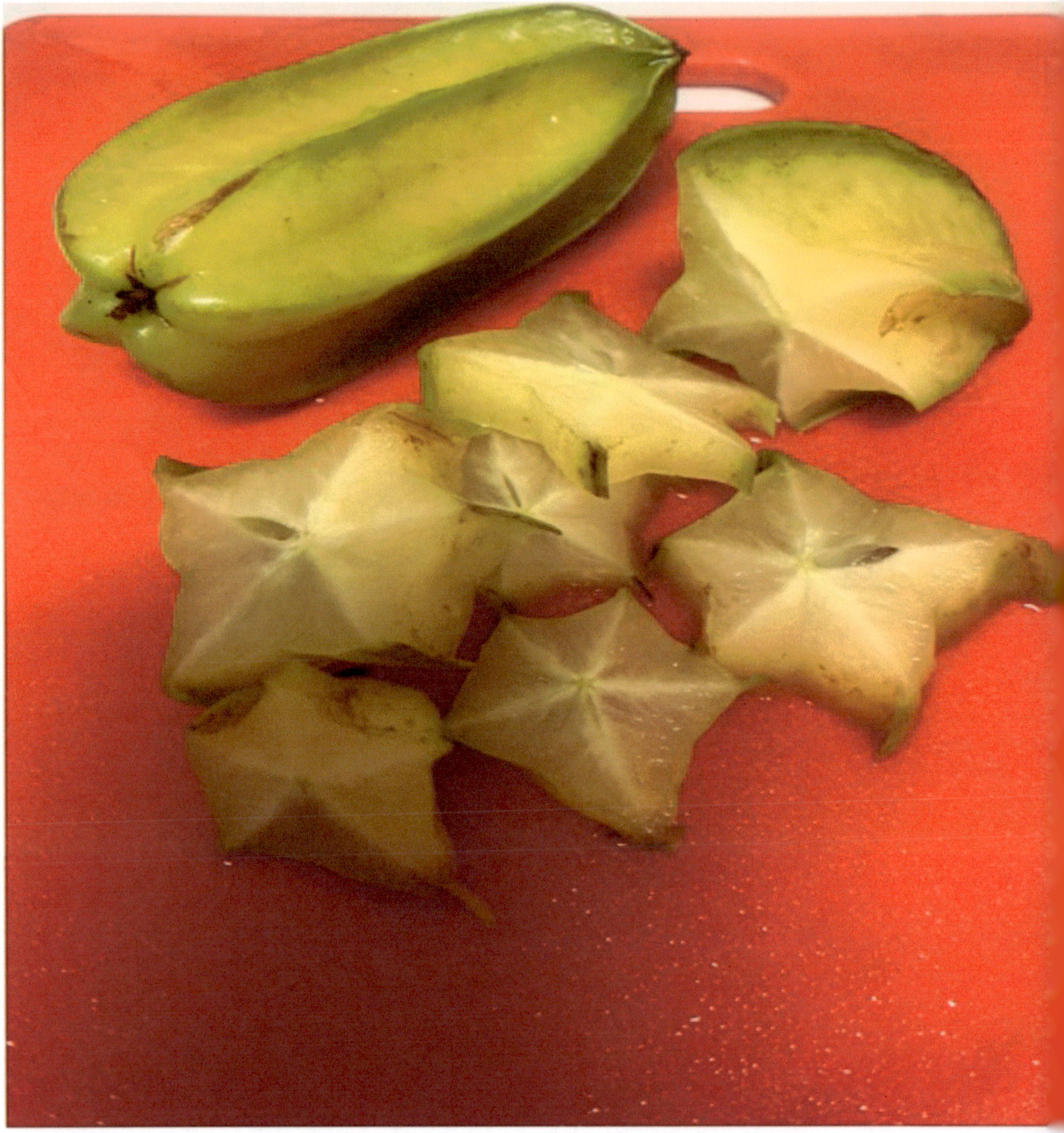

Kiwifruit

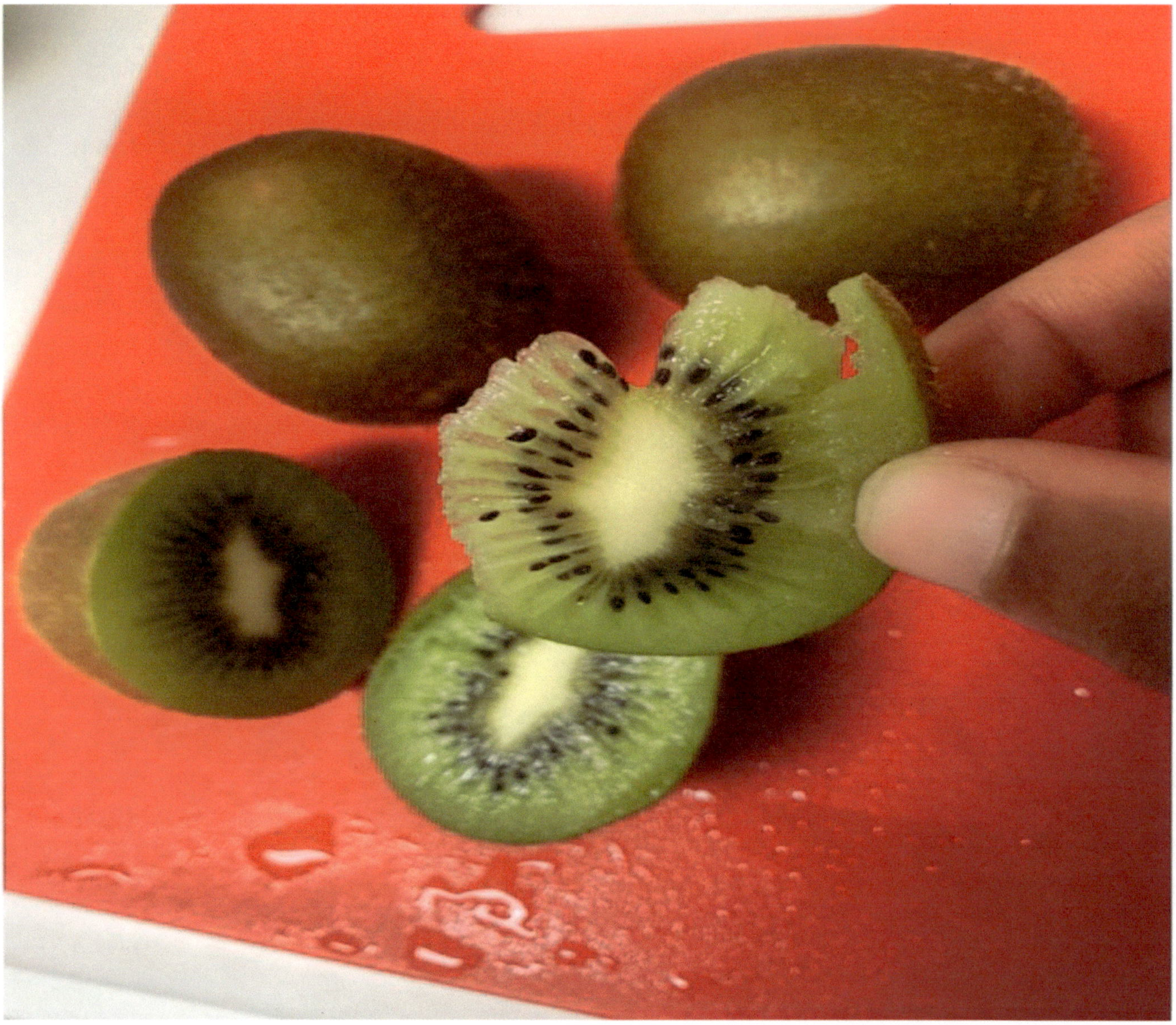

Made in the USA
Monee, IL
05 November 2026

67380853R00045